Developing

WINNING
ATTITUDE
&
MINDSET

C000136260

Other Works by Allistair McCaw

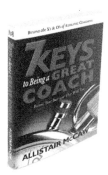

7 Keys to Being a Great Coach

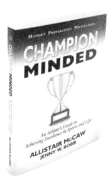

Champion Minded

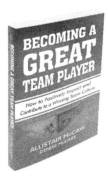

Becoming a Great Team Player

The most important decision you can make in life is the attitude you choose to adopt.

Developing a
WINNING
ATTITUDE
&
MINDSET

50 Ways to Positively Transform
Your Career, Your Relationships and Your Life

by
ALLISTAIR McCAW
DENISE McCABE

DEVELOPING A WINNING ATTITUDE & MINDSET – *50 Ways to Positively Transform Your Career, Your Relationships and Your Life*
Copyright © 2020 Allistair McCaw

All rights reserved. No portion of this book may be reproduced, stored in a retrieval system or transmitted in any form or by any means, without the expressed written permission of the publisher.

A reviewer however, may quote brief passages in a review to be printed in a newspaper, magazine or journal.

First Edition – April 2020

Published by Allistair McCaw

Allistair McCaw
M

www.AllistairMcCaw.com

ISBN: 978-0-578-59026-4

Library of Congress Cataloging-in-Publication Data

Category: Self-Improvement, Leadership, Lifestyle, Mindset

Author: Allistair McCaw | McCawMethod@gmail.com

Co-writer and Editor: Denise McCabe | www.McCabeEditing.com

Cover Design and Layout Graphic Artist: Eli Blyden Sr. | www.EliTheBookGuy.com

Printed in the United States of America by Printer:
A&A Printing & Publishing | www.PrintShopCentral.com

Disclaimer

Limit of Liability/Disclaimer of Warranty: While the publisher and author have used their best efforts in preparing this book, they make no representations or warranties with respect to the accuracy or completeness of the contents of this book and specifically disclaim any implied warranties of merchantability or fitness for a particular purpose. No warranty may be created or extended by sales representatives or written sales materials. The advice and strategies contained herein may not be suitable for your situation. You should consult with a professional where appropriate. Neither the publisher nor the author shall be liable for damages arising herefrom.

Contents

SECTION 3

Attitude Police for Negative Thoughts

SECTION 4
Self-discipline

SECTION 5
Role Models

SECTION 6
Empathy

SECTION 7
Perspective

SECTION 8
Embrace Change

Introduction

First, let me commend you for picking up a book focused on developing a winning attitude and mindset. This simple act says that you are already interested in transforming your career, your relationships and your life. Look around and you will see that people who have chosen a more positive attitude and mindset generally live longer and enjoy a happier and more successful life than those who view the world through a negative lens. The attitude and the mindset you choose will either push you forward or hold you back. What do you choose?

For more than 25 years I have had the privilege of working with some of the highest achievers in the world – Fortune 500 CEOs, stars in the music and entertainment industry and world-class athletes – and I can tell you that their success is not the result of more knowledge, more experience or mystic superpowers. It is the result of their relentless work ethic and commitment to consistent daily action. Under performers lack such consistency in their habits and routines; high performers, on the other hand, maintain this consistency. In addition, they have chosen a sharp focus on attaining excellence; they have chosen to stay disciplined in order to achieve their goals and the life they wish to live. What do you choose?

I often hear people complain that they don't have the right qualifications or experience, that they don't have the right looks, the right education, enough money, etc. They find every excuse in the book to justify the fact that they aren't where they want to be. Truth is, excuses get you nowhere, and no one really wants to hear your constant complaints. You see, everything you ever wanted is on the other side of the negative excuses you keep telling yourself. One of my favorite maxims about positive choices is this: *The average do it sometimes. The good do it most of the time. The great do it all the time.* What do you choose?

Marcus Aurelius, the Roman Emperor and stoic philosopher, once said, "You have power over your mind – not over outside events. Realize this, and you will find strength." I'd like to add that you will also find self-empowerment. I believe that each and every one of us has the potential to achieve way beyond our wildest dreams. Through a change in attitude and mindset, I have seen contenders become champions and non-starters on a team become regular starters. I have seen college scholarship applicants, job applicants, and people with far less experience and skills be selected over others who may have had the perfect qualifications on paper, but fell short in what mattered most – their attitude and mindset. What do you choose?

I have written this book because I want you to *know* that you have the unlimited potential to become more than you could ever have imagined, and how to do it. You can become unstoppable. But for this to happen, you will first need to reexamine your attitude and mindset. You must be ready to make some changes – some big, some small, some scary, some exciting. Throughout the pages of this book, I will share with you the lessons I've learned about human behaviors and how strongly your attitude and mindset influence your relationships, your career and your life. You will see some of the most important points more than once. I will also share stories and examples from my own experiences as well as those of others.

I have structured this book in bite-size chapters for you to read, reflect on and act on. You may choose to read it from start to finish, or to mull over just a few chapters a day. Whatever your approach, I encourage you to equip yourself with a yellow highlighter or a pen, and mark the quotes or parts that stand out for you. Then you can refer to them easily and share them (whether by talk, text or social media) with your friends, family and colleagues.

Section 1, Master Your Mindset, emphasizes the fact that your most important relationship is with yourself. To develop a winning attitude and mindset, you first have to take control of your thoughts, because they become your reality. Avoid people who bring you down, and instead spend time with those who, like you, are fueled by a greater purpose and who inspire you. But remember to be your own greatest fan and to never lower your standards to please someone else.

Section 2, The Power of a Positive Mental Attitude, reveals that your mental attitude is one of the best kept secret assets you possess. Have you noticed that those who have a positive mental attitude bring positive energy, too? Work toward this: Be all in. Let your smile brighten others' days and attract them to your positivity and potential. Believe in the possibilities. Celebrate your wins, even the small ones. Embrace your failures: They teach you more than successes do, and they let others know that your self-confidence means that making mistakes is not an embarrassment to you.

Section 3, Attitude Police for Negative Thoughts, conveys the importance of having in your head your very own police squad that stops negative thoughts in their tracks and replaces them with positive ones. Instead of comparing yourself with others, focus on being the best YOU you can be. When you find yourself in a high pressure situation, instead of viewing it as a threat, think of it as an opportunity to shine. Let go of the past and get rid of old ideas that are holding you back. Let optimism set you up for success.

Section 4, Self-discipline, stresses the fact that no long-term success can be achieved without self-discipline – intentional and consistent commitment to your goals. Give yourself the edge by following my 5% theory: Whether your team is in sports or at work, give the extra 5% that others don't. Others may have more in the way of natural gifts than you do, but do not let anyone outwork you. Be known as the person who always does more without having to be asked or prompted. Remember that self-discipline could just be the most important attribute to creating the lifestyle you want.

Section 5, Role Models, provides some great examples of people who have inspired me or set examples of upbeat approaches to life, in spite of various obstacles. Paul, the barista left to do the work of three people, still managed to brighten everyone's day. Oliver, the tennis coach and cancer victim, maintained right to the very end the positive attitude he advised others to have. Jose, the grocery bag packer, Nick Bolletierri, the tennis coach, and Babette Hughes, the novelist, all in their 80s, work with enthusiasm every day. Richard Branson, Walt Disney, and J.K. Rowling, at different times in their lives had to employ their winning attitudes and persevering mindsets to overcome others (who should have known better) who told them they weren't good enough. These three achievers must really have enjoyed the last laugh!

Section 6, Empathy, explains that people with winning attitudes and mindsets tend to have higher levels of emotional intelligence and empathy; they are more in touch with who they are and how they think. They appreciate the importance of strong relationships with others and letting them know their value. People with a winning attitude and mindset come to accept that they have flaws, and then to accept that others have flaws, too. They are better able to understand others, and the reasons why they think, act and behave as they do. Those who gain these insights build and nurture relationships, displaying a higher level of kindness toward others. People who choose self-awareness and healthy control over their emotions are far likelier to get along with others and to succeed.

Section 7, Perspective, shares a habit I consider a game changer in my life: the principle I call GAS – gratitude, appreciation and self-reflection. Practicing this simple regimen each day will help you identify your greater purpose and vision, and live them to the fullest. Because life is unique for each person, no one has all the answers. Respect others' ideas so that they will respect yours. Embrace life with happiness and gratitude every day.

Section 8, Embrace Change, underscores the fact that those who are stuck on their old ideas – their "that's the way things have always been done around here" attitudes – are inevitably making themselves irrelevant. Closed minded people who don't embrace change will be left behind. Redesign your life; recommit yourself to excellence, and outdo yesterday. Add forgiveness to your life. Consciously make a list each day of two or three things you are grateful for. These practices will impact your life in amazing ways. Make it your habit to grow and improve consistently each day.

Most people love the idea of being great – until it's time to carry out what greatness requires: consistency. Consistency means dedicating yourself to a task, activity or goal, every day. It means staying disciplined and engaged even when you don't now feel like it, every day. Despite good intentions, most people cannot keep this up. Either they lack the discipline or their purpose is just not strong enough. But consistency is how people with winning attitudes and mindsets succeed, every day.

Just as with deciding what clothes you are going to put on today, your attitude and mindset are choices. To win in life, you first need to win in your mind. It all starts there. What you think is connected to all that you do, and the attitude and mindset you choose can be the difference between achieving your best life and falling short.

The truth is, developing a winning attitude and mindset takes a lot of work, and it doesn't happen overnight. The way you think today is an accumulation of all that has occurred in your life – your upbringing, beliefs, trials and tribulations, ups and downs, joys and pains, highs and lows. As with mastering any new skill, forming a winning attitude and mindset requires hours and hours of dedicated and consistent practice. And it's worth every minute! As you develop these skills, you will discover that you've become more likeable, interesting, inspiring, thoughtful, appreciative, empathetic, energized, positive, engaged and alive – to name just a few of the side benefits. Wow!

A really wonderful future is waiting for you. All you have to do is realize the importance of holding yourself accountable: Stick to what you said you were going to do and stay disciplined, especially when you'd rather not. I don't believe for one second anyone was put on this earth to be ordinary. I believe that you were made for greatness. I believe that you have everything you need inside you. What are you waiting for? I encourage you to implement some of the lessons in this book, let go of limiting beliefs and become unstoppable. Choose to commit consistently each day to developing and growing the attitude and mindset that set you up for happiness, success and most importantly, fulfillment. Choose to transform you career, your relationships, and your life. Trust me, your future self will thank you.

– Allistair McCaw
February 2020

SECTION 1

MASTERING
YOUR MINDSET

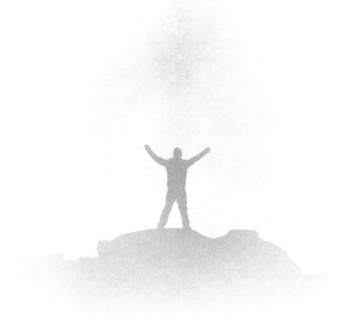

Chapter 1

Your Most Important Relationship Is with Yourself

I believe that the key to happiness is found in building long-lasting relationships – relationships that are meaningful and rewarding. But there is not one of greater importance than the one you have with yourself. As Belgian fashion designer Diane Von Furstenberg noted, "The most important relationship in your life is the relationship you have with yourself. Because no matter what happens, you will always be with yourself."

One certainty is that you can't expect to live a positive life when you have a negative and limited mindset, much the same as you can't have a healthy relationship with yourself if you aren't appreciating and acknowledging the goodness in your life on a daily basis.

When you wake up in the morning, what is your inner voice saying to you? What about throughout the day or before you go to sleep? Is it positive or negative, empowering or disempowering? The truth is that how you talk to yourself matters more than you think. What you say to yourself shapes how you speak to others, how you act and how you live. What is on the inside always flows outward and influences others. The thing to remember is that most of us aren't naturally positive, especially when it comes to how we see ourselves. Most of us seem to gravitate to being negative about ourselves. But remember that we get to choose how we will be.

Our self-image comes down to self-talk. One of the most powerful forms of self-talk comes in the form of mantras. I like to use them with the athletes I work with. The word mantra has two parts (in Sanskrit): "man," *thoughtfulness with zeal*, and "tra," *to protect*. So, when you say something to yourself like "I love to be challenged" or "I am great at this skill" over and over, it starts to become a part of you, a deeply ingrained belief. Unfortunately the opposite is true as well. If you tell yourself negative things like "I can't do this" or "I'm not good at math," you will eventually believe it. Whatever you continually tell yourself becomes a part of your subconscious mind. Over time, you begin to become what you keep telling yourself even if it was never true at the beginning.

Your self-talk is the biggest part of your day. In fact we talk to ourselves more than we talk to anyone else. It's wise to talk nicely! The only way to get respect and admiration from others is to stop disrespecting yourself and your potential. It's time to acknowledge who you are and who you want to be. You must remind yourself that you are good enough, that you have what it takes, and yes, that you matter and can make a difference in this world.

Sometimes in life you come across people who are nasty or unkind. What you very often find is that these people have an unhealthy relationship with themselves. They play the victim and view the world as unkind, unfair and selfish. These feelings might have arisen from situations or events that happened in their past – negative experiences, unhealthy environments, toxic relationships or just having a poor self-image. They try to bring others down to their own level of unhappiness. Have as little to do with them as possible.

For better or for worse, people come and people go throughout life. You will gain and lose friends, partners and other people along the way. But no matter who walks out of your life, remember this: Never ever lose yourself. It's something I learned the hard way several years back when I lost myself after a breakup. This is the most important thing: Learn to love yourself when you feel unloved by those around you.

Everything changes when you begin to love yourself. You see the world and others from a much better place. However, the outside changes only when the inside does. Become a powerful source within yourself that attracts better. The more you love who you are, the less you seek validation and approval from others. Remember – if it is everyone else you are trying to keep happy, the only person who won't be happy is you.

The brain believes what you tell it. When you feel gratitude and appreciation for the things in your life, no matter how small they might seem, you nurture positivity with yourself and with others. When you learn to love yourself and accept yourself, the ability to build and have great relationships with others becomes stronger because you attract what you reflect. The better person you become, the more likely positive people will be attracted to you. To attract better, treat yourself better. Start transforming your attitude and mindset. Start upgrading your habits. Start being more positive.

People with a winning attitude and mindset accept themselves for who they are and where they are right now. They are grateful for who they are while working on being a better version of themselves. They don't beat themselves up over things. Be proud of your progress and keep taking steps forward no matter how small. You will eventually reach your full potential. You'll look back on the days you thought you'd never make it, and you'll smile and be proud that you never gave up on yourself. Yes, believe it, everything in your life is about to change, but only if you are willing to take the steps to change. It starts with the relationship you have with yourself and your self-talk.

Helpful Hints to a Better Relationship with Yourself

- Practice gratitude and appreciation

- Be good to yourself

- Refrain from judging others and yourself

- Learn to see the good in yourself and others

- Forgive yourself and others

- Love and accept who you are right now

- Let go of the past; it's gone

- Self-reflect daily; write things down

- Wake up each morning and tell yourself how awesome you really are!

———————————————

You are only one thought and decision away
from changing your life.
Appreciate and talk kindly to yourself.
You can do it!

Chapter 2

Your Thoughts Become Your Reality

When you take notice, you can see that people's attitudes determine their outcomes. The most successful people, be it in the corporate world, in the sports world or in life, are those who believe in the possible. They are positive thinkers and have a winner's attitude and mindset.

If you want better outcomes and results, be willing to reevaluate and improve your attitude and mindset. Put a stop to all the unhelpful negative thoughts, and consciously replace them with positive thoughts. Find the mantras that speak to you, or create your own. If you think you can do something, you will find a way to make it happen. Visualize yourself as the person you want to become and be that person right now. If you want to be the CEO of a successful company or a great athlete, start walking, talking, thinking and doing like one – not just acting, but *doing* like one. It's easy to come up with excuses not to do something. It's harder to push yourself to do what it takes to become the person you want to be. But it pays off big time in the long run. Think about someone who worked really hard to become successful. Do they think the hard work was worth it? That's a very big Yes!

What happens when you don't choose a more positive mental attitude? A negative mindset delivers you negative outcomes. A pessimistic mindset limits your incredible potential. If you are always thinking about what could go wrong, chances are, it probably will. Want to know one of the biggest limiters to success? It's overthinking negatives. You must factor them in, but dwelling on them leaves no time to conceive fresh ideas or strategize executing them. You attract what you think. For better or worse, your thoughts become your reality.

Have you ever been really excited about an idea, project or something you've thought up, only for someone to give you all the reasons why it won't work? It's happened to me. It is incredibly difficult to deal with, especially when that someone is someone close and important. I was so excited to share my ideas with this person, but within a matter of a few minutes I was given all the reasons why it would never work. I wasted many opportunities by not taking enough action. Now obviously not all your ideas are going to excite everyone, but those who have achieved great things in life have looked past the naysayers and operated with an attitude of "I can and I will."

Here's the thing. You don't need 99 reasons why something won't work; you need just one why it will work. Don't be limited by small or negative thinkers. They are why it's important to surround yourself with the right people. They are not necessarily those who agree with all your ideas, but people who can see both sides of the equation, people who aren't afraid to give you the truth. Be around people who inspire you. Go to environments that expand your mind. Your life is your choice. Don't depend on someone else to say, "Hey, you know what, I think you did great" or "you didn't do so great." You are the one to decide whether you did great or not, and you are the one to decide what your next path is. Don't let somebody else decide that for you.

Contrary to the popular saying, the world doesn't belong to the dreamers; it belongs to the doers. Those who take action. Those who aren't afraid to fail or be mocked. Those who aren't afraid to be rejected. They are the people who keep going. If you really believe in something, then go for it. What have you got to lose? So what if you make mistakes and endure failure along the way? Every mistake takes you one step closer to success. Every successful person who has gone on to achieve great things has had to endure rejection, failure and disappointments. You might not know when or how bad, but they surely did. Remember that nothing worthwhile in life comes easy. When you have a winner's attitude and see the reasons why something can work, then amazing things can happen.

Your attitude is the foundation of your success, and you get to control it. It in turn controls your actions, and they in turn prompt other people's reactions to you. If you choose to start with a positive attitude, many other aspects in your life will fall into place in positive ways.

In much the same way, if you choose to start with a negative attitude, many aspects of your life will fall into place in negative ways. Negative attitudes come from thinking negative thought patterns over and over until they become part of your subconscious, part of your personality. They become habitual. They lead to failures and disappointments.

"So how do I get control of my thoughts and become a positive person?" I hear you ask. Well, like anything else, it takes consistent commitment. It also involves changing certain beliefs. How? You need to be more aware of what you are thinking and saying to yourself on a daily a basis. Sometimes we aren't even aware of all the negative little thoughts that pass through our heads. Pay attention to them.

The first step is to catch yourself in the act of being negative. The words we say to ourselves on a daily basis can either be incredibly constructive or incredibly destructive without us even being aware. Those subconscious thoughts become our beliefs, and our beliefs become our reality. When you catch yourself complaining or being negative, actually say to yourself "Stop!" Then consciously replace the thought with something positive. For example, if you say to yourself, "I'm terrible at math" you could replace it with something like "I'm getting better at math." You might not get it 100% right the very next time you attempt something, but what you are doing is priming your brain to think positively.

Here's the truth about positive people and those with winning attitudes and mindsets: They also get negative from time to time. The main difference is in how quickly they can eliminate and change those thoughts.

Be more aware of your thoughts and what you say to yourself. When you practice this simple exercise, you begin being more positive until it becomes a habit. You are replacing an old unhealthy practice with a new healthy one, much like replacing drinking soda with drinking more water. Remember that you get what you think.

A winning attitude and mindset produce
more than just positive thoughts:
You become your thoughts.
Make sure yours are self-empowering and
compelling every day.

Chapter 3

Avoid the Energy Vampires at All Costs

Have you ever felt completely exhausted, like the energy has been sucked out of you when you are around a particular person or particular people? I'm pretty sure you have. I certainly have. Energy vampires are everywhere. Usually this kind of person likes to complain about everything under the sun. When they walk into a room, you can immediately feel a difference in that space. These energy vampires are experts at being buzzkills.

Energy vampires may sabotage much of their own success and happiness by moaning and complaining all the time. And even when they have some success, they are happy undermining others. So, with this in mind, the process of developing a winning attitude and mindset involves separating yourself as far away as possible from these folks. When I speak about this at events and workshops, often someone in the audience asks something like "But, Allistair, isn't that kind of selfish and negative? Shouldn't we be helping people like that become more positive?" I think my answer surprises them at first when I say no, because here's the thing: We all get to choose our attitude. These energy vampires, like you and I, have a choice to either be positive and uplifting or negative and gloomy. We can definitely be the example for others, but in the end it's up to them to decide.

Look, we all go through stuff; we all have our challenges and we all have endured failures and disappointments. Life can be hard, but we all have a choice about how we are going to live today and beyond. You can choose a winning attitude and mindset, but you can't change someone else's attitude; only they can change that. When their choice is negativity, stay away from them!

I've discovered over the years that not only do some people not want to change, they actually enjoy being negative and miserable. It gets them attention from others and it gives them control over others. I'm sure you can already think of someone who is like this. They would rather be gray and gloomy than be excited and inspired – it's the truth. These are not the kind of people you want to be around. They suck up useful energy that you could better use to improve yourself.

Energy vampires feed off your emotional, or psychic, energy. You will discover that the people who display energy vampire traits generally lack compassion, empathy, and emotional maturity. Energy vampires are not necessarily bad or nonproductive people. In fact one could even be a friend, a family member, a work colleague, a teammate, or even a romantic partner. They are concerned only about their own well-being.

Word of warning here! Energy vampires are often attracted to people with winning attitudes and those who exude a positive energy. The reason is that they love to suck that out of you for their own benefit. Unfortunately, if you're a highly empathetic and compassionate person who doesn't know how to say no or set boundaries, it's very likely that you're surrounded by energy vampires right now!

Energy vampires are everywhere. They love to pull you down to their level to make themselves feel better. They are the kind of people who thrive and survive on gossip, negativity and other people's shortcomings. They are the kind of people who, if you are working on improving yourself and you're making progress, will tell you that you've changed. And your answer to that? "Thank you! Thank goodness I've changed!"

Take stock of who you have in your life right now and who you surround yourself with on a daily basis. Are they energy providers or are they sucking the life out of you? Don't let the vampires steal your greatness and your opportunity to live your best life. Remember, a winning attitude involves separating yourself from the energy vampires.

5 Ways to Distance Yourself from Negativity

1. Unfollow and delete negative people and platforms from your social media

2. Don't spend a lot of time watching or listening to negative news on TV or radio

3. Distance yourself from the energy vampires

4. Don't entertain gossip

5. Don't get into discussions about politics or religion

In order to create a more relaxing and rewarding life, take the steps necessary to get rid of the energy vampires in your life. Make it your practice to avoid them at all costs.

Chapter 4

Winners Hang with Winners

Winners learn to avoid people who have little purpose, ambition or direction. People with winning attitudes and mindsets surround themselves with those who are like-minded and fueled by their greater purpose. They are people who are going places. When you are in their company, you will notice that the conversation is different. People with winning mindsets and attitudes don't waste their time talking about people; instead, they spend their time talking about their goals, dreams, ambitions and strategies. In addition, they don't dwell on problems, but rather on answers and solutions.

What I'm talking about here is who you invest your time and energy on and with. The people you choose to call your friends are a reflection of what you value and stand for most. Be selective about who you spend your time with. I would far rather have two or three close friends I can trust, than a hundred friends I can't. It's quality over quantity. However, that doesn't mean you seclude yourself from others, as it is gratifying and rewarding to know and be friendly with many people.

Let me ask you this: Have you ever paused to take stock of the people you have in your life? The great motivational speaker and author Jim Rohn once said, "We are the average of the five people we spend the most time with." Think about it – when we are around people for an extended period of time, we begin to eat like them, dress in a similar style, go to the same places, listen to the same kind of music or watch the same sports. Our language and even the words we use start to be the same. In time, we become who we hang out with, without even realizing it.

If you don't want negativity or pessimism in your life, then stop hanging around negative and pessimistic people. If you want more than average, stop hanging out with average people. If success is important to you, stop hanging out with people who have no ambition or only criticize your efforts. If kindness is important to you, stop hanging out with unkind people. Your friends and peer group are a great reflection of – and influence on – you. This is a very important point that I stress to the groups I speak to, but it is especially important for kids and young adults in school. Hanging with the wrong person at just one wrong moment can devastate your future. Choose wisely.

When you decide to let go of certain people in your life, those who aren't contributing to your goals, ambitions, and happiness, it can initially be painful and uncomfortable, but in the long run it is liberating and transformational.

Get with people who are on the same mission as you or those who have achieved what you desire to. If you want to see why someone has been incredibly successful in the field you are in, spend time with them, observe their habits and routines and listen to their words. There is a caveat here. While it's ideal to be closely surrounded by positive, supportive people who want you to succeed, it's also necessary to have your critics. When you surround yourself only with yes people, those who are afraid to tell you the truth, you are still surrounding yourself with people who limit your potential of becoming your best self. We need to remember that constructive feedback and criticism – hearing the good, bad and the ugly – are important for our personal growth. We don't improve from hearing only the things we want to hear, so we need to surround ourselves with people who are not afraid to tell us what we need to hear and who have our best interests at heart.

———————————————

Surround yourself with people who inspire and encourage positive change in your life.

Chapter 5

Become Your Own Greatest Fan

If you don't back yourself, love yourself, value yourself and appreciate yourself, then why would others believe they should? It's you who gets to call your value in this world. Here is the honest truth: There is no one quite like you. In fact, if you could see yourself through other people's eyes, you might realize just what an awesome specimen you really are. You were made for greatness, remember? Why is it that we often don't see the amazing qualities in ourselves?

Jay Shetty, the Indian English influencer said, "When nobody else celebrates you, learn to celebrate yourself. When nobody else compliments you, then compliment yourself. It's not up to other people to keep you encouraged. It's up to you. Encouragement should come from the inside." Jay's advice certainly resonates with developing a winner's attitude and mindset.

I'll admit it; I haven't always been my own greatest fan. I'm pretty hard on myself at times. In fact, it's something I have recently sought professional help for. I wouldn't call myself a perfectionist, but rather someone who always viewed good as never good enough. Come to think about it, great wasn't great enough either. Even though I'd exude confidence on the outside, deep down inside I was never satisfied. For example, after achieving something I'd worked so long and hard for, like writing a book or completing a marathon, I just never took the time to enjoy the accomplishment or applause because instead I'd already be onto the next goal, the next book or the next project. I remember listening to an interview with Toto Wolff, the Mercedes Benz Formula 1 boss, who mentioned that he suffered from this dilemma. Even after his team won a Grand Prix race or even a world championship, he said he'd never take any time to enjoy the moment and, in fact, moved right onto planning the next race or world championship.

For me, this not stopping to smell the roses all became too exhausting, and a while back, I felt things had to change. My health was up and down, and my moods began to change. I began to feel demotivated and discouraged. I realized that I wasn't living up to having the right mindset. That is when I started to make some changes in how I was viewing my successes and accomplishments.

Having healthy relationships with others is important, but, as I've noted, none more important than the relationship you have with yourself. It's all starts there. Yes, real authentic happiness comes down to the relationship you have with yourself. Now understandably, you might be thinking, "Oh wait, here's this guy writing books on positivity, attitude and mindset, but he struggles with it himself." Yes, it's true. That's exactly the reason why I felt compelled to share my journey with you and share what many others experience. No matter how perfect life might look from the outside, we all struggle with things, especially our self-image and attitudes, from time to time.

We all have flaws and parts of ourselves that we don't like. Furthermore we all have made mistakes and maybe have some regrets, but to live a life of joy and greatness, we have to be willing to let go of the past, accept our current position and move into the future with positivity and optimism. We must embrace the mindset of being happy just doing our best. I'm a strong believer in seeing any experience in a positive light and dealing with the lessons it can teach us, no matter how awful it seems at the time. That's why getting to know yourself and reconnecting with who you are, rather than the person you may usually mask yourself as, is a worthwhile investment in both time and effort, like I did when I realized the need to make a change. Becoming your own greatest friend involves congratulating yourself on the struggles you've overcome. You know that you can master the ones in the future.

Being your own biggest supporter, friend and coach in whatever you do is probably one of the best things you can and will do for yourself. In fact, it's a necessity in developing a winner's and attitude and mindset. Daily we are bombarded with negative thoughts, doubts or distractions, and it seems so easy to talk or break ourselves down. The destructive and self-defeating self-talk is nothing but wasted energy and unhelpful to our well-being. The feeling of not being good enough or not ready for something isn't helping you in any way. This kind of inner dialogue with ourselves keeps us from moving positively into the future.

Winners talk to themselves like winners. They are honest with themselves, but they don't berate themselves. When you talk negatively to yourself, you instantly sabotage your own success, no matter how far you've come or how well prepared you are. Besides, you already have enough competition in this world. Why become your own toughest opponent when you can become your own greatest inspiration, motivator and source of strength?

Understand that true confidence comes from first loving yourself, accepting yourself and believing in yourself – accepting all your flaws *and* appreciating all your strengths. Remember, it's important to keep the positive promises you make to yourself and never compromise. Maybe it's time for you to stop getting in the way of your own happiness and success. Learn to invest in growing the relationship you have with yourself. You are more than worthy, believe me. Everything you need is already inside you. Just get to know yourself better. Let go of the past; understand that the past is history. Today, make a commitment to how you are going to be moving forward.

In a world where you can be anything,
have the courage to be you –
accept your flaws and move forward
with courage and positivity.
It's time to become your own greatest fan.

Chapter 6

Soar with the Eagles

When I was growing up, my father often reminded me that "you can't soar with the eagles if you hang out with turkeys." Of course, he was referring to the fact that the levels of success you attain are related to the company you keep. Life is too short and precious to be around anyone or anything that doesn't first of all make you a better person. To be a winner in life you need to surround yourself with winners. People who want to go far in their lives have people around them who are also on a mission go far in theirs. It's easy to determine who the people with a winning attitude and mindset are because they are the people who are talking about their goals, dreams and aspirations. These are the people who are excited about their future and what lies ahead.

Developing a winner's attitude and mindset involves surrounding yourself with people who get you out of your comfort zone and challenge you. That's why it's important not to spend time with people who are okay with being complacent. Spend time with those who inspire you. These are the people you want to be around.

Another thing that you'll notice about people who have a winning attitude and mindset is that they don't spend time around drama or negative energy. They are very selective about their time and energy. They see their energy as precious and protect it against every negative thing or person as much as possible.

Winners act like winners, look like winners, think like winners, compete like winners, prepare like winners, communicate like winners, commit like winners and live like winners. They are never arrogant or over-confident, but instead are humble and hard-working. Winners don't need to tell you how invested they are in improving themselves; their actions speak for them. Winners take daily consistent action. Even when they don't feel like it, they do the work. They are driven because of a deeper sense of purpose.

Surround yourself with loving people who bring out the best in you, instead of wasting time with people who cause you to compromise. Spend time with people who push you to rise higher. Spend time with people who support your dreams, goals and vision. Spend time with people you can learn from. Spend time with people who make you laugh. Spend time with people who let your inner child out to play on a regular basis. Spend time with people who will be there on the dark days, not just the bright ones. Spend time with people who are good for your mental health. Spend time with people who encourage you to grow.

Make room in your life for people who care enough about you that they hold you accountable. Find people who can even sometimes discipline and motivate you without belittling you. As you grow older, you realize it becomes less important to have more friends and more important to have real ones. Cutting toxic people off from your life doesn't mean that you hate or dislike them; it just means you respect yourself enough to remove negativity and stress from your life by not having to deal with them anymore.

Spend time with people who are

Able to get things done	Humble
Appreciative	Inspiring
Authentic	Not judgmental
Consistent	On a mission
Empathetic	Positive
Generous	Purposeful
Going places	Selfless
Grateful	Sincere
Happy for others' success	There for you
Helpful	Uplifting
Honest	

---

*People you choose to have around you
should consistently bring out the best in you,
not the stress in you.*

Chapter 7

Never Lower Your Standards

P eople with winning attitudes and mindsets don't lower their standards for anyone. One of the main reasons they are able to do this is that they have gotten over worrying about what other people might think. It's not that they don't care what others think, but rather that they care more about where they are going and what they are doing. They understand that it's their journey, their life, and they accept that others won't always understand or go along with that.

We shouldn't be limited by what other people might think of us. I believe that our greatest potential already lies within us, but it can sometimes be our own limiting mindsets and attitudes that stop us.

It's often our ego that counterintuitively gets in the way of our greatest achievements and learning potential. It's funny, but if you think about it, we aren't worried only about what other people think if we fail, but also about what they think if we succeed. In many cases, what we then do is either give up on our amazing ideas and aspirations or we simply lower our standards to suit and fit in with those around us. We want to stay humble, so we become afraid to shine and stand out, scared that we might be viewed as pompous or arrogant. So, with that in mind, why are you trying so hard to fit in, when you were born to stand out? Why are you holding yourself back from becoming your best self? Who cares what others think? Maybe it's time to get over that hurdle and adhere to the standards you want for yourself. Maybe it's time to embrace the life you were meant to live.

Developing a winning attitude and mindset involves keeping the highest of standards. You are not responsible for the opinions or reactions of others. Some will feel threatened by your standards, and that's OK. That's their problem, not yours. Don't let the bad habits of others, or their laziness, weak character or lower standards influence or rub off on you. Keeping the wrong company is a huge limiter to your success and ability to have a winning attitude and mindset. It is like riding a bike with a flat tire; it won't get you where you want to go. You need to be your own person. You need to set your own personal bar high and never lower your standards for anyone else. If others are offended, that's not your problem. If they are offended by your standards, then let them be the ones to live with lower ones – and the consequences.

Your values and personal standards define you. People who are on a mission to better themselves or achieve greatness understand that it's much more than a 9-to-5 job. A few years back, I was talking with an athlete who had won two Olympic golds in swimming. We were chatting about what separated the very best from the near best. At the top of her list: "your daily standards and not compromising for anyone." Wise words indeed.

Pause for a moment and think about this: How and how much are you influenced by the people you spend time with? Take a few minutes to think about that. What do they bring to you? Do they bring out the best in you? Are you inspired and energized by them or do you feel that you are drained by them? Here's another question: Do you find yourself compromising your values, making excuses, procrastinating or lowering your personal standards just for them? One of the key aspects of what separates the successful from the unsuccessful lies in the standards they hold themselves accountable for. When you are pursuing an outrageous dream or goal, a fake friend will give you every reason why you can't do it. They will try to pull you away from what you are trying to achieve because they don't want to feel left behind. Again, that's not your problem and you aren't responsible for that either. A real friend will give you every reason why you should and can do it. A real friend will be the one who checks up on you and keeps you accountable.

What about romantic relationships? There can be nothing worse than being in a relationship that is toxic or one that is holding you back from becoming your best. One of the most important decisions you can make in life, if not the most important, is choosing the person closest to you and who you choose to spend your time with. You will more than likely adopt many of the habits and traits of your partner over time. If you're involved in a relationship right now, ask yourself if that person is making you better. Is that person challenging you and encouraging you to succeed? Does that person uphold or even better your own standards?

People with winning attitudes and mindsets succeed because of the higher standards they keep for themselves. Stay humble, stay hungry, stay grounded. Keep your standards high and be a person who lives with integrity and dignity. And remember that at the end of the day, if you're not proud of who you are and the way you choose to live your life, little else matters.

_____

One of the most important decisions
you can make in life is
in choosing the person
you decide to spend the most time with.
Their habits, attitude and mindset
will be contagious.
Choose wisely.

THE POWER OF A POSITIVE MENTAL ATTITUDE

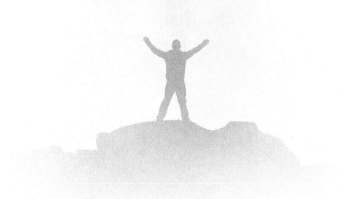

Chapter 8

A Winner's Attitude
Brings Much Opportunity

People often ask me how I am able to put up with so much traveling and flying around the globe for my job. First, I see it as a privilege to do what I do. Second, traveling gives me the opportunity to shut down the phone and either read, research, or reflect. It's what I call my 3 Rs.

I like to take opportunities to chat with strangers. In fact, I've had some of my most enjoyable conversations with strangers. They teach you so many things you might otherwise never know about. On a flight to New York last year for a speaking engagement, I struck up a conversation with a gentleman seated next to me.

I learned that this gentleman was the owner and CEO of a very well known company that owns a chain of health clubs and spas. We discussed what great team players look like and how to find the right person for leadership jobs. He said something incredibly insightful. When he or his team was out and about, be it in airports, restaurants, visiting other clients, and in fact, anywhere, they were always on the lookout for people who could one day be potential employees.

When I asked him what he looked for, he replied, "Someone who gets along with people and someone who exudes a great energy and attitude." Those for him were the most important traits. In fact, he told me that about 7 years earlier he had hired a young man (we'll call Mark), who was only 23 years old and had little work experience, to work as a duty manager in one of his health clubs. He had met Mark while on vacation when Mark was working as a waiter and barista at his favorite coffee shop. What impressed him most was the already evident high level of emotional intelligence and ability to interact with his customers on a daily basis. He recalled the time an irate customer was rude to Mark after she received the wrong coffee. Mark apologized, smiled and brought the correct order to her, on the house. Seven years later Mark was the head of operations on the east coast, overseeing 85 managers nationwide. What did the CEO see in Mark? The attitude of a winner.

We often go places where we are greeted by less than enthusiastic employees or workers who hate their jobs. Unfortunately what these people don't see is the potential and opportunity they have every day to meet new people and display their abilities. You see, opportunity is everywhere – if you choose to bring your best attitude and energy. You might not like what you are doing now, but, like everything else, it is only temporary.

Attitude is a choice, and if you don't bring a good one, you can't expect to get those "lucky" breaks and opportunities. In fact, do you want to know who usually ends up with those lucky breaks in life? No, it's not always the most talented or skilled. It's the people who put themselves in the position to get them – the people who choose the right attitude. The people who will do more than just what has been asked of them. The people who come up with solutions faster and stay optimistic no matter how dire things are. These kinds of people understand that they might not be where they want to be right now, but by bringing a winner's attitude and mindset, they put themselves in the best position to succeed and get ahead in life. They are aware that among the people who see them on any given day could be the one who can improve their life forever.

Young Mark understood the bigger picture. Mark knew that his job at the coffee shop was temporary, but that it gave him the platform to meet people, expand his network, and then go on to greater things. No matter where you are right now, no matter how much you dislike you job or what you do, be like Mark and see it as a great opportunity to meet new people and expand your network. Mark had a choice. Either he could be miserable and bitter about his current circumstances, or he could be excited and optimistic about what was next to come.

You never know who's watching. You never know when or where that next great break or opportunity might come. That's why consistently keeping a winner's attitude, a positive energy and an optimistic mindset is the best thing you can do in life.

———————————

With a winner's attitude,
opportunities can come to you
that you never could have imagined.

Chapter 9

Adopt an All-in Attitude

A winning attitude is about being all-in. When I speak to teams or groups of people, I like to remind them of this: Regardless if you are in a company, on a sports team or in a relationship, you are either all-in or you're not. You can't achieve true success or happiness if you choose to just dip your toes in the water or put in the work only when you feel like it. Being all-in is about committing yourself to the highest of standards and bringing your very best self each and every day. Not always easy, I know, but achieving great things was never meant to be easy.

I may seem like a very positive person who always stays motivated, but I'll be the first to admit I don't always wake up in the morning excited and leaping out of bed. That's why I give myself a pep talk, practice gratefulness and sometimes have a personal attitude management meeting with myself.

Not long ago I had the privilege to interview Bob Bowman on my podcast. Bob is the longtime coach of the most successful Olympian ever, Michael Phelps. In fact, Bob is one of the most successful coaches in sports history – lauded for his intense personality, incredible dedication to his athletes, and ability to nurture talent in athletes who have the heart and drive to win.

I read Bob's book *The Golden Rules – Finding World-Class Excellence in Your Life and Work.* I couldn't put it down and finished it on a flight from Fort Lauderdale to Dubai! In it Bowman lists his 10 success principles, the second of which advises, "Be all-in!" This principle presses on the fact that no matter how talented you are, without the right attitude, you won't succeed or reach your full potential. Remember that a negative mind will not contribute to a positive life.

During our conversation on the podcast ("Champion Minded" podcast on iTunes, episode 46, season 1), Bob made it clear that the right attitude matters more than you may think. He believes that the highest crime you can commit is to bring the wrong attitude to a training session. Competition is in fact all about being present and bringing your very best attitude and effort to that moment, regardless of how you feel.

Bob noted that "positive people fully invest in the process and face challenges and adversity far better than those who are closed minded and negative." In Bob's training sessions there are high standards, such as no complaining, blaming and moaning. Jokingly he added that those who want to complain are welcome to go underwater and do it, so no one has to hear them!

Bob is a coach of excellence. "An all-in attitude can turn long shots into legends. Use positive energy to go after your dreams. Double down on what it is you want, allowing no room for doubts or negativity. Be enthusiastic about your vision and take enthusiastic action. Be committed to forging ahead even when you feel like getting out."

———————————

Take this lesson from one of the world's greatest coaches and motivators. Be all-in every day!

Chapter 10

A Winning Attitude Involves Energy Management

The human brain and body are like a battery, and like a battery need to be recharged from time to time to have sufficient energy to run. We have only so much energy in a day, so it's important for us to learn how to properly gauge it. In developing a winning attitude and mindset, it's impossible to go full out all the time. If you are a participant in the rat race, constantly pressuring yourself to do more and more can eat you alive. Just like athletes who train hard and must learn to rest adequately in order to perform at their best, if you are pushing your limits and maximizing yourself every day, you can't go full out all the time. You can't sprint through a marathon.

I've learned this the hard way a few times. Because I'm too often pushing to the limit, I've burned out a few times in my athletic career and in my coaching and consulting career, too. We often don't know where the line is until we cross it. As recently as a couple years ago I again landed in what I call the red zone – empty. I depleted my tank. I took over 100 flights, was in 26 countries and 43 cities. I spoke at 94 events and consulted over 600 clients, some I keep in daily contact with. On top of that I wrote my third book together with Denise McCabe, *Becoming a Great Team Player*. Last but not least I ran over 1700 km (1056 miles) in a year. Toward the end of the year, I began to feel my energy and attitude deplete. When you are tired, mentally and physically, it's difficult to give others your best, no matter how hard you try.

I believe that energy is foundational to success. The energy you have (health). The energy you give (service to others). The energy you bring (attitude). The energy you share (relationships). The energy you allow (standards). The energy you save (rest and recovery). And most important, the energy you don't (or do) permit in your life (drama and negativity). The most important factor to our energy and overall performance is our health. I'll refer to the example of athletes, but the principle is true for everyone. In order to perform at an optimum level, they first need to find the balance between hard work and rest – what sports science calls metabolic recovery. If athletes push too much without getting adequate rest, they get either injured or ill as a result of overload. It's a very fine line. Likewise, it is important for everyone, whatever field we may be in, to better balance the delicate ratio of work to rest.

Recently I posted on my Twitter account (@allistairmccaw) that I believe more than 70% of coaches, teachers, and leaders are burned out. People in service industries are taking care of others' needs first. The long hours, the weekends away, the traveling and then of course taking care of families. So often I see people in these positions working on empty. You can't take care of others if you don't first put on your own oxygen mask.

A few weeks ago, I was traveling with an athlete in Europe. The trip was supposed to be six weeks long. However, after three weeks on the road, and balancing other work-related responsibilities, I felt my energy and performance decrease. I also felt my moods and irritation levels increase, which is not the standard I want to have when working with clients. Being in better touch with myself (let's call it personal competence) I knew I had to take a step back. So I flew home for a few days to recharge; I returned fresher, revitalized and stronger. The athlete and I finished that part of the season strong and with a winning attitude. This is an example of energy management and knowing thyself.

Know your limits and catch yourself before you fall. You can't expect your car to keep running if you don't check that battery regularly. Having a winning attitude and mindset really involves consistently paying attention to the condition of your whole self, both mind and body.

———————————

In order to consistently bring your best, learn to manage your physical and psychological energy well.

Chapter 11

There's Power in a Smile

Have you ever noticed that confident and happy people smile a lot? It's not that they don't have the same challenges and struggles as everyone else; it's just that they choose to see life through a different lens. As a kid, I didn't smile that much. I was always serious about things. One of the major reasons was that I was embarrassed about a gap between my two front teeth. I was so self-conscious, I kept my mouth closed and usually wore a poker face. I was often told to smile more, but I didn't.

After having my teeth fixed, I learned how to smile again. But it was an effort, and sometimes still is. I suppose you could say my face muscles had been programmed to not smile. I had to retrain my smile muscles. Did you know it takes only 12 muscles to smile and 113 muscles to frown? I was wasting a lot of energy back then. Don't let this happen to you!

When you smile, you invite and attract more people toward you. You become much more approachable and tend to open up conversations that lead to relationships. In addition, smiling improves your attitude. If you have any doubts, next time you feel down, smile and think positive thoughts and see what happens.

Even in a tough situation with another party or dealing with an angry customer, an appropriate smile relaxes the mood and tension. Smiling also raises your confidence. It makes you feel more competent and self-assured in any interaction.

I encourage you to try this: Just for one day smile at every person you meet or pass by. They might think you're crazy, but that's okay. For example, when you walk into work, smile at the members of your team, ask how they are and even share a compliment with them. Smiling ignites positive energy and positive attitude. People start to perform at a higher level because their self-esteem has risen. They will respond to you in more positive ways. Try it for just one day and see what a difference it can make.

Here's another important thought. You never know how much someone else might need your smile and a compliment today. They cost you nothing but are actually priceless. They can give others hope and even change their lives. Your smile shares your energy and your winning attitude, and draws them out in other people. As I like to note, people may forget what you said, but they remember how you made them feel. When you make them feel good about themselves, they will feel good about you.

When you are about to greet someone, make sure you first have a smile on your face. Again, no cost to you, but invaluable to someone else. You may never know how much that one smile or compliment meant to their day or even their life.

Smile and you will find the world smiles back at you. The opposite is true as well – but who wants to think about what that looks like!

Here are my 5 Ss when approaching or meeting someone:

1. Smile on approaching that person.
2. Shake hands (always look them in the eyes).
3. Share a compliment (it can be anything, even "I love your shoes!").

4. Share your contact information (have a business card ready).

5. Send a follow-up within 48 hours (a text or an e-mail to say that it was a pleasure to meet them).

When you meet someone, instead of thinking, "What can this person do for me?" smile and think, "What can I do for this person? How can I help them?"

Use your smile to change the world;
don't let the world change your smile.

Chapter 12

You Never Know Who Is Watching

We live in an age where we can no longer do things that go unseen or even unheard. Today there are iPhones, video cameras and eyes everywhere. We have to be on guard now more than ever because we never know who is watching us.

Many years back I was working in Sicily where I was in charge of the sports operation division of a hotel. Part of my duties included making sure that all our facilities and equipment were ready for the visiting teams of athletes who came from all over Europe to train in the off-season. They were Tour de France cycling teams, endurance swimmers, world-class triathletes, runners, mountain bikers, etc.

One evening a gentleman approached me while I was packing up equipment after a practice session. He introduced himself in a thick German accent as Gunther, and he invited me for a coffee to discuss a proposition he had for me. When we met the next morning, he explained that he owned a few sports facilities and other successful companies in Germany and Switzerland, and asked if I'd be interested in the possibility of heading up a very large sports performance facility in Berlin, Germany.

Gunther went on to explain that part of the job description for this project would be to work with some of the best trainers, coaches, doctors and athletes from Europe. I was blown away by the offer, and asked him where or how he had heard of me. His reply was that he really didn't need to see my credentials, qualifications or accolades as he'd been observing me for a few days working with the coaches and athletes around the hotel, and he had also asked around about me. What he had seen and heard was enough for him to know that I was what he was looking for and what he needed.

Gunther said that he had been able to tell by my attitude, energy and work ethic that I was the person he wanted to head up his exciting sports performance project. He said he was very impressed that I was able bring a positive attitude and demeanor to work every day. I thanked him and promised I'd get back with my answer within a few days. In the end, I didn't take the job due to my decision to continue competing for a while longer, but it certainly opened my eyes to how the real world works.

Today we are made to think that the certificate or letters behind our name are everything, but they aren't. Now please don't get me wrong. I am not saying that you don't need a good education – you do. I am saying that your attitude will get you way further in life than your qualifications or degrees. When you are able to bring a winning attitude and mindset to your day, you are able to open doors and opportunities that can lead you to bigger and greater things in life -- not only in your career, but in the quality of your relationships, too. And trust me, building relationships is huge if you want to get ahead in life and in your career.

Always be at your best. Always bring your best – regardless if you feel like it or not. You never know who is watching. It could be a potential sponsor watching your practice, it could be a coach looking to recruit, it could be a business owner looking for a great partner or employee, or it could even be your next amazing romantic partner in life!

You are your own brand and walking billboard every time you step out the door. That brand value is dramatically increased when it brings a winning attitude and great energy to those around it. The way you act, look, talk, walk and behave reflects who you are, and developing a winning attitude includes all these things.

Be respectful and well mannered. Hold doors open for others. Say hello and thank you to strangers. Shake hands.

These are the small things that make a big impression on others. You never know – that person watching could be the person who changes your life for the better!

Always bring your best and always be at your best because you never know who is watching.

Chapter 13

Believe in the Possibilities, Not the Probabilities

I've just woken up in my hotel in Marseille, France. It's May 8, 2019. I'm still buzzing. Last night was the second leg of the Champion League Football tournament, the most coveted trophy and biggest club tournament in football. The match was between the mighty Catalan giants Barcelona and my beloved Liverpool. Liverpool had to win 4-0 on the return leg at Anfield. Possible? Highly unlikely according to many experts, especially against the current best team in the world. Adding to the difficulty of the task, Liverpool was without their two standout players, Brazilian Roberto Firmino and Egyptian Mo Salah.

The British betting company Betfair had the odds at 50-1 against Liverpool. However, being an optimist, I still believed a miracle could happen. We had come back from a 0-3 deficit against AC Milan in the 2006 Champions league final to win, so why not?

On the morning of the game, I went down to breakfast at the hotel wearing my Liverpool shirt. A gentleman standing behind me in the line asked, "Do you seriously think that your team is going to win tonight?" My response was that I believed 100% in it, to which he replied, "Good luck with that! Although crazy things happen."

Well, crazy things did happen. Liverpool pulled off the impossible and won 4-0. This meant that they would go through to the final in Madrid on June 1.

Here is one distinct quality I've noticed in the most successful people or highest performers I've worked with and been around: They are total optimists. They believe anything is possible. No matter what the odds are against them, they believe they can and will succeed. What we understand about optimism is that it comes down to having a deep inner belief.

Before the match, Liverpool's leading striker, Mo Salah, was seen wearing a t-shirt at the grounds that boldly advised, "Never Give Up," and the mighty Reds, as Liverpool is known, never did give up, even against the very best team in the world with a three-goal deficit. This is a really great lesson. A winning attitude involves belief. Not just some belief, but a committed and all-in belief. A real winner's attitude is about staying optimistic and believing in what others might view as impossible.

The next morning I listened to the post-match comments on Spanish television from TV pundits and fellow coach Jose Mourinho. The experienced Portuguese mentioned that this incredible comeback really came down to German football manager Jurgen Klopp's own belief and the belief he had instilled among his group of players. Belief was the key.

Looking back to my school days, I was told by my high school cross-country coach to "never give up and always believe that it's possible." In every race I participated in, her words were present in my mind. Thank you, Caroline Vorster! Those simple words have stuck with me throughout my life and have helped me achieve things I never thought possible. Guess what? They can do the same for you. I'm here to tell you today that when you adopt an attitude of optimism and belief, amazing things can happen in your life. When you put in the work, take control of your thoughts and block out the doubt, you can achieve the impossible, just like Liverpool did.

Optimism is a choice. Winners understand the power of their mind and choose to feed it positive thoughts and images constantly. Next time you are doubting yourself or an outcome, no matter how impossible it seems, take the path that gives you a greater chance of success. Change your mindset from "I can't" to "I can."

And for the record, Liverpool went on to win their sixth European champions trophy three weeks later in the final against Tottenham Hotspurs, 2-0. Always believe. Never give up!

Champions are champions not just because of their skills, but also because of their ability to stay positive under adverse situations and keep an attitude of optimism and belief.

Believe in yourself every day;
great and surprising things will happen.

Chapter 14

Celebrate the Small Wins

I'm often asked, "Allistair, how do I build self-confidence?" A simple question, right? I like to use this analogy: Confidence is a like a brick wall. Every day you are either building it up or breaking it down. When you are able to recognize all your small wins on a daily basis, you add bricks to your wall. When you focus only on what's going wrong, you break it down.

Each day offers us the chance to build our self-esteem and confidence. Without even realizing it, we perform daily activities that are actually small wins in the bigger picture; for instance, waking up early to exercise or read, eating a healthy breakfast, doing a good job on a project or presentation, making a great play at practice or even hydrating more throughout the day. Even compliments are victories. For most of us, these small victories go unnoticed, but they actually deserve our attention.

Another great practice is to self-reflect each evening and write down what you did well that day in your journal. Writing things down and seeing them strengthens your belief and heightens your motivation. Taking notice and focusing on the daily small wins are essential steps in the process of growth.

Unfortunately, from a young age, many of us have been hardwired to notice our mistakes and shortcomings. Looking back at my life, I know that I was always pretty hard on myself about every little thing I didn't do well. What I didn't do enough of was notice the small things I was doing well or allow myself to celebrate any victories. In fact, even after completing my first book, a lifetime goal, I didn't take a day off to celebrate the achievement. Instead I was on to writing my next book. In retrospect, I wasn't contributing to my happiness or confidence. Only later did I realize what a game changer it is to focus more on appreciation and catching myself doing things right. When I began to build my wall of confidence, I saw better results.

How I wish I'd realized this earlier. The lesson: *It's never too late to start building your wall of confidence.* Through this process, you will be able to train your mind to see the good in things more often and recognize the small things and blessings that occur on a daily basis. The result? Way more confidence and motivation, which will result in way more appreciation, fulfillment and joy.

If you are one of those people who allow themselves to celebrate only final outcomes or bigger moments, then not only are you losing out on the enjoyment of the process, but also you are missing out on what it's all about – the journey. When you celebrate today, you bring yourself joy and positivity; when you look back on it in later years, you will realize that remembering the times celebrating yourself brings you joy and positivity yet again. A double life win.

Don't wait to celebrate your greatness only when the bigger wins or outcomes happen. Take the time to notice your small wins so as to appreciate them and yourself, too.

To develop a winning attitude,
make it a habit every day to recognize
and celebrate the small wins – and yourself.

Chapter 15

Failure Teaches Valuable Lessons

A baby learning to walk keeps falling over and over again, but that kid never thinks to himself or herself, "You know what, guys? Screw this. Maybe this walking thing isn't for me." Instead the baby keeps trying until this walking thing is mastered. The truth is that a baby can be one of our greatest teachers in persistence – falling, getting up, falling, getting up and trying again.

Something I've learned in working with some of the greatest athletes and high performers in the world is that they see failure differently from the rest. These successful people keep a positive attitude, not allowing setbacks, failures or mistakes to hold them back. They are forward minded, stay persistent and keep their eyes fixed out the windshield, and not the rearview mirror. They see failures and mistakes as vital lessons in their growth.

I believe that not being willing to learn from failure, or avoiding it, stems from our ego. We're afraid of losing our reputation, our image, our social status, and our influence. One thing I know about every successful person who has achieved excellence is that they have taken risks, knowing that they might fail.

What you'll find with these high performers is that they are willing to get out of their comfort zones and do what others aren't willing to do. They are willing to fail and look stupid in front of millions because they have learned to tame their ego. These people are willing to put themselves out there more than the rest, understanding that when they do this, although their chances of failure are bigger, in the long run, the rewards are greater. And therein lies a defining reason why these people succeed – they are willing to take more shots and miss than those who are afraid to. In fact, it reminds me of a quote from the legendary ice hockey player Wayne Gretzky, who noted, "You miss 100% of the shots you don't take."

When we do only what we know how to do, we don't learn or evolve. We stay in a comfort zone where nothing grows. And if we are not growing we are not getting better. Having a winning attitude and mindset is all about trying to get better every day in every way possible. What winners see differently when it comes to failure is that when they fail, they are simply one step closer to getting it right. With a growth mindset, winners see failing as a step closer to succeeding. Failure provides answers, but only if we are open to receiving them. It is something that should be viewed as a hurdle rather than a roadblock. Successful people aren't discouraged or derailed by failure. They know that every worthwhile goal carries some element of disappointment.

For some, failure is viewed negatively, as an opportunity to feel sorry and complain, a reason and an excuse to give up. But those with a winning attitude and mindset don't see failure as the opposite of success; they see it as a part of it. They don't beat themselves up about failing; instead they get straight back onto their horse again. They see it simply as a challenge to be overcome, and in the end, a learning opportunity.

The truth is that the difference between a stepping-stone and a stumbling block is found in the attitude you choose. As Zig Ziglar said, "Remember that failure is an event, not a person." Don't be afraid of failure; it's your greatest teacher.

———————————————

Ever tried? Ever failed? No matter.
Try again. Fail again. Fail better.

– Samuel Beckett

Chapter 16

Vulnerability Reveals Inner Confidence

Some of my most meaningful relationships, and ones that have lasted still to this day, have come from being able to stay vulnerable. Unfortunately, and admittedly, I was pretty late to this game, but applying this concept even to those outside a close circle has been a game changer for me.

Think about the people who others choose to connect with most. They relate to those with imperfections, and not so much to those who seem perfect. My own approach and message in speaking engagements has changed over the years from what might have looked like the perfect way to consult with clients or train world-class performers to being more open about my failures and vulnerabilities. The difference this has made in my ability to connect with my clients and audiences on a much deeper and more meaningful level has been extraordinary. I believe it reveals inner confidence.

At first speaking about my fears, shortcomings, and failures scared the living daylights out of me. Today I'm proud that I can be more vulnerable and open to speaking about my many failures and mistakes. Fact is, standing up there and telling everyone how amazing your life is or how you achieved a lot of success might be inspiring to a select few, but to the majority it isn't relatable or realistic. People buy into the product only when they buy into the person first; that is, they can relate to you in a more humane way.

The thing is this: People don't know who you are until you learn to be vulnerable. Vulnerability involves letting go of the ego and learning to laugh at yourself. Being able to laugh at yourself tells the world that you are confident and secure in yourself. Give yourself permission sometimes to look stupid or silly. In fact, I will open a speaking engagement or presentation with a story about a major mess up I've had or a time when I felt like an idiot. This allows the audience to immediately feel like they have a connection with me. Because, guess what? *We all screw up!* It's human.

Being vulnerable with others opens up another level of relationship. In fact, just yesterday I had lunch with a great coach in Boca Raton. Kyle and I have known each other for some time professionally, but we have never sat down and really gotten to know each other. After a bit of chitchat about the industry, etc., the conversation changed to another level. He shared some things that were personal and difficult for him. We were willing to become more vulnerable and share a few struggles going on in our non-professional lives. A 30-minute meeting turned into an hour and a half. I left feeling refreshed and as if I'd been to a therapy session. The truth is that talking is therapy, but we men especially don't do it enough. Women do a far better job at this. It felt great to share more of my life and to hear about his. In fact, ego can be our greatest enemy, something that can inhibit our progress and be our greatest obstacle. I'm grateful for that meeting, for that deeper conversation and for Kyle.

Yes, being vulnerable feels uncomfortable at first, but remember that it's when we get uncomfortable that we grow. No growth has ever occurred in a comfort zone. As best-selling author Brene Brown says, "Choose courage over comfort." Of course, you must be careful about who to trust, but when you allow yourself to be vulnerable with the right people in the right way, you begin to set yourself free.

Vulnerability is not a weakness;
it is a great measure of strength.

ATTITUDE POLICE FOR NEGATIVE THOUGHTS

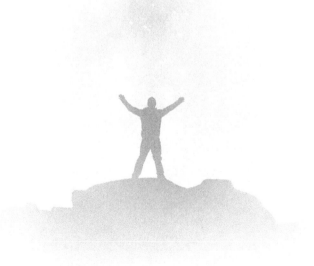

Chapter 17

Let Your Attitude Police Arrest Your Negative Thoughts

S taying positive and keeping a winning attitude isn't always easy. Each day we are confronted with many challenges which can test our patience and mood. Just yesterday I was flying back from Madrid, Spain, to Fort Lauderdale, Florida. After a very long journey I was greeted by an extremely busy customs hall with lines winding up and down for what looked like miles.

Not a problem, I thought to myself. After ten years I had finally received my green card and was pretty excited to be entering the United States for the first time as a permanent resident. I was sure I didn't need to join that long line for non-US residents. However, after I showed my card, the airport steward told me that I did indeed have to join the long queue of non-residents. I felt my anger and frustration build up immediately. My expectations had been crushed.

My first thought was "how can this be?" After I joined the long and winding line, I immediately started to grumble to myself things like "this is pathetic" and "I can't believe this." I continued to think these negative and unhelpful comments, but – surprise! – they didn't speed up the line or make any difference at all. It was then that my "attitude police," as I like to call them, showed up, blue lights and all. My attitude police are my internal attitude management task force who appear when I start to moan, groan or complain about things. I have trained myself to quickly stop in my tracks when I think things that aren't helpful to my mood and energy.

So standing in the line I started to replace these negative and useless thoughts with positive ones like "how lucky am I that I have a green card!" and "this is a great opportunity to pull out the book I'm reading and make use of my time." Instantly I began to feel my energy pick up. I started to appreciate the good things I had going for me.

As with any skill, mastering your mindset requires discipline. Without supervision, our minds are ruled by random and often negative thoughts. If we allow negativity and what I like to call garbage to take up residence in our heads, then that is what's going to take over our subconscious. The more you train your mind to look for the good and stay positive, the more empowering and helpful it will become. You will live each day in a better frame of mind, and others will be more likely to be receptive to your ideas and opinions.

I am often asked, "Allistair, how do I stay more positive?" It's a great question, because it's hard to be positive when, for example, someone or something really annoys you. Dial up your attitude police. The first step is to catch yourself being negative. The second step is to stop yourself cold and replace negativity with something positive. Your attitude police to the rescue.

---

*One of the best ways to become
a more positive person is to catch yourself
in the act of thinking negatively.
Each day aim to be on guard,
and change your negative thoughts
into positive ones.*

Chapter 18

Manage Your Morning Attitude

I'm a morning person, but that doesn't mean that I wake up each day fired up and ready to change the world. I mean, I'd love to, but it's not exactly realistic. Besides, after years of extensive travel I think my body doesn't know if it's in the southern or western hemisphere anymore, never mind what time it is.

One strategy I use to get myself going in the morning is to have a personal "attitude management" meeting with myself. "A.m." (ante meridiem) may be the abbreviation for morning, but for me it stands for "attitude management." I make sure that by the time I start my commute to work, I have checked my attitude. I prime myself for performance by making sure I am in a positive frame of mind.

One thing that gets me into a winning frame of mind is starting the day with gratitude, focusing on what and who I'm thankful for in my life. I try to be original each morning by finding different things to be grateful for. Also, I try to visualize how I'd like my day to be. If I have meetings, I visualize the setting and the person or people I'll be with, and the outcomes I'd like us to achieve. I can't tell you how many people have said to me, "I can't believe how upbeat and positive you are in the morning!" I reply, *"It's all about your attitude!"*

Another thing I do in the morning is to have no radios or televisions on. I have heard that the ratio of negative to positive news is 9:1. Is that a good way to start your day? If you have stayed at some hotels in the United States, you will also relate to TV in the breakfast area blaring all the negative and depressing news. I usually either move as far away as possible or take my earphones and listen to a great podcast.

Ever heard those irritated, impatient and horn blowing people in the traffic? Sometimes I wish I could stop them and share my message. When we are angry in traffic and complaining about everything from slow drivers to red lights, we are just creating negative energy that drains our whole well-being. And while we are on the topic of commuting, instead of turning on the radio, listen to a podcast or some light, easy music to put you in a calm and relaxed mood.

Important: Protect your energy. Choose carefully what you listen to, what you watch, who you follow on social media, who you surround yourself with and the environment or surroundings you're in. Run from negative energy. Run from negative people. Remember, that you are responsible for the energy you put out and put up with.

I'm a firm believer that your attitude in the morning controls your energy. If your thoughts are negative and unhelpful, for example, you might say to yourself, "I feel so tired." Then guess what? You will feel tired! Your words are incredibly powerful and persuasive. Now I'm not saying that you don't get tired because, of course, we all do. What I am saying is that you aren't helping your energy when you're telling yourself negative things. Remember that your body hears absolutely everything the mind thinks and says. Think, act and talk positively and with enthusiasm, and you will feel the difference, believe me!

I prepare my attitude for the day and like anything else, and the more I practice this, the better it becomes. I purposefully get my mind in the game, just like an athlete getting ready to compete or a dancer getting ready to perform. Now, there are days when I'd prefer to stay in bed with the pillow over my head, but I know that's not going to take me closer to my goals and my greater vision and purpose in life. I understand that I owe my best to those who trust me to serve or consult them.

In fact, one of the most important contributors in my career successes is consistency in my attitude and energy. I've learned that clients will pay more for the value and attitude you bring to the table than for just your skills. Of course, having the skills is important, but you can find those anywhere. Possessing a winning attitude both in your career and in your life is the key to success. Fact is, most people who pay you for your services don't really care how you are feeling or how badly you slept. They pay you for your ability to perform at a consistently high level with a great attitude. One example I tell those in the fitness industry, such as personal trainers and coaches, is that clients come to you more because of your energy than your exercises.

Remember that each morning requires us to have an attitude management meeting with ourselves. A consistent winning attitude starts right there.

Start every day with the mindset of
"I get to" instead of "I have to."
This is how you set yourself up for success.

Chapter 19

Comparing Yourself to Others Is a No-win Game

One of the things that hold many of us back from acquiring a winning attitude and mindset is comparing ourselves to others. It causes us to focus on someone else's gifts, talents and purpose instead of our own. It's what happens when we are focused on success versus excellence.

There was a time before Instagram, Twitter, Snapchat, etc. – pre-Photoshop days when people's images were rarer and more accurate. Today we live in an era of social media bombardment and are fed images of the perfect bodies, new cars, great looking guys and girls with the perfect lives. Or so we are led to believe. What happens is that we tend to compare our lives to everyone else's highlight reel and doctored photos. We begin to ask what's wrong with us – and it's a trap.

Comparison is the thief of joy. It's a no-win game. I'm not telling you to get off social media, but if you want to be happier, then maybe quit following those people who keep posting how amazing their butt or new car or boat is. If that's what you value, then you can expect to be playing no-win and "I feel worthless" games. Truth is, there will always be someone more beautiful, fitter, richer, smarter, taller, more knowledgeable, whatever. And if there isn't, believe me, you'll search until you find them. That's how most of us are wired. Stop.

While success is often measured by comparison to others, excellence is all about being the best we can be and maximizing our gifts, talents and abilities to perform at our highest potential. To be our best, we must focus more on pursuing our own excellence. We must focus on being the best we can be and realize that our greatest competition is not someone else but only ourselves. Anyway, what's the point of comparing when all of us are traveling a different journey?

An important point to remember about this is that it's not only about where you are going; it's about who you are becoming along the way. Since comparison with others is a no-win game, doesn't it make sense that the only person worth comparing yourself to – and improving upon – is the person you were yesterday? Focus and work on that.

I can't remember where I heard this, but think about it. We spend our first 20 years worrying what people think about us. Then we spend our next 20 years swearing that we don't care what people think about us – but of course we do. Then we spend the next 20 years realizing that they weren't even thinking about us in the first place.

Focus also on learning to be grateful for what you already have. If you are reading this, the chances are that you have food, shelter, running water, and access to education. Congratulations, because you are ahead of the vast majority of the people in the world. Take a minute right now and think of five things you are grateful for. People who focus on cultivating their gifts and their strengths are happier and more successful than those who dwell on compensating for their weaknesses. They don't compare themselves to others.

In the final analysis, do you think that you will wish you had spent more time comparing yourself to others?

Five Regrets Expressed by the Dying

1. I wish I'd had the courage to live a life true to myself, not the life others expected of me.
2. I wish I hadn't worked so much.
3. I wish I'd had the courage to express my feelings.
4. I wish I had stayed in touch with my friends.
5. I wish that I had let myself be happier.

Why compare yourself to others? No one in the entire world can do a better job of being you than you.

Enjoy the journey.
Let go of comparisons and
embrace your uniqueness.

Chapter 20

Attitude Trumps Ability

In episode 56 of my Podcast *Champion Minded*, I got to talk to the inspirational Richard Whitehead. Richard is a double amputee runner, world record holder in the 200 meter and double Paralympic gold medalist (at the time of this writing). Richard's feats also include running 40 marathons in 40 days.

Like I do with every guest on my podcast, I asked him what it means to be champion minded. Richard replied, "Being champion minded is all about attitude beating ability every time." Richard, a fantastic speaker, spoke about the importance of having a winning mentality and attitude in life. When you listen to Richard, it's easy to tell that he's a can-do kind of guy. I don't think the word *can't* is in his vocabulary. Richard is more human doing than human being, someone who sees no limits to what he can do. The more he is doubted, the more he gets motivated and focused.

Richard believes that a person's attitude can be their greatest tool in achieving success in life. He doesn't waste time on the naysayers or critics. He believes in putting in the work, staying patient and always believing in himself. Richard is a perfect example of having a winning attitude and mindset.

I remember when I was competing in my seven-marathon and seven-half-marathon challenge back in 2016. It was marathon number three in West Palm Beach. That day, like most days in Florida, was an incredibly hot 92°F (33°C) and humid. This just six days after I had run a marathon in Minneapolis in freezing temperatures of 11°F (-12°C)! I was around 25 kilometers into the race (15 miles) when my body started to resist and fight against me. I remember thinking to myself, "How am I going to even finish this race, never mind four more marathons?" It was at that moment that my personal attitude police took over. I got hold of my unhelpful thoughts and changed them immediately. It was from there I was able to replace those self-defeating thoughts with more helpful and empowering ones. I began saying things to myself like "every step is one closer to my goal" and "you got this, Al, you can do it." As simple as it sounds, I began to feel better when I changed my weak attitude to a winning one.

I've worked and consulted with many people, not only in the sports world, but in other high performance industries, and I have seen how attitude trumps ability time and time again. I have seen people who had all the opportunities in life be overlooked due to either poor attitude or inferior work ethic. Just last week, I was speaking to a friend who runs one of the most successful IT companies in California. When we spoke about hiring and what he looked for in his team, he emphasized that attitude and personality will always be the main two areas in hiring. Of course, he looks for the right skills and competence, but the ability to get along with others, work together and have an attitude of positivity and gratitude are necessities.

Richard Whitehead also counseled, "Enjoy the moment, and enjoy the people around you." Powerful advice about what really matters in life. Follow it, go into all you do with a positive attitude, regardless of your ability, and you can find yourself moving ahead of those with more ability but less positivity.

If you believe that life has limits, you will always struggle. Let go of that limited mindset, and know that if you make it a habit to think more positively, life will be more positive.

Ability is what you're capable of doing.
Motivation determines what you do.
Attitude determines how well you do it.

– Lou Holtz

Chapter 21

Winners View Pressure as Opportunity

According to former Olympic diving gold medalist Greg Louganis, there are two kinds of athletes or performers when it comes to approaching competition. Louganis describes the two perspectives as "energies." The first type of person enters the competition arena and interprets the energy as a threat and as pressure. The second type of person enters the competition arena and interprets the energy as excitement, opportunity and fuel.

These two types of people are separated by only one thing – attitude. In my experience working with high performers, Olympic medalists and world champions in their chosen disciplines, I have seen firsthand how those who perceive that energy as pressure and stress succumb on most occasions. And conversely, I have seen those who have chosen to perceive that energy as exciting and an opportunity to display their skills succeed and thrive.

The athletes and performers who see that energy as stressful are more outcome and result focused – ends ultimately not under their control. Those who see that energy as invigorating are more process and in-the-moment focused. Even though they want to win and succeed, they don't fear outcomes as much as they see them as opportunities to learn and grow. They have an attitude and mindset of always trying their best, but not fearing the outcome.

One such person who comes to mind is tennis player Lloyd Harris of South Africa. I started working with Lloyd in December 2018. At Wimbledon 2019 he drew the Swiss master Roger Federer in the first round, a daunting prospect for any player on his Wimbledon main draw debut! Lloyd had never played on Centre Court before. He had never played at Wimbledon before. He had never played a top-10 player before. He had never played Roger Federer before. He didn't have any of Federer's 20 Grand Slam titles or 107 matches of Wimbledon experience. He didn't even have a single tour-level win on grass to his name. But there are upsides to playing your idols, too.

Instead of complaining about what arguably is one of the toughest first round opponents, Lloyd thought to himself, "Damn, what a great opportunity to show the world what I can do. What's more, I know everything about him. I've seen him play 1,000 times in my life. And he's never seen me play. That's a good start, I guess." Sure, he felt a little nervous, but he walked onto the center court with a winner's mindset. To the surprise of many, Lloyd even won the first set, giving Roger reason to be nervous. He eventually went down in four sets, but he used it as a fantastic learning experience.

Here is another point that is important to remember: Every athlete feels nerves. The ones with a champion minded attitude and a winner's mindset see those nerves as a sign of readiness and excitement for what's to come. If you're an athlete or someone who gets nervous, then great, because even the best of the best get nervous, too! I have seen it firsthand in the locker rooms of Grand Slam events – tennis players such as Federer and Nadal looking nervous before going out to play. I've seen some of the biggest names in rugby, football, golf, squash, badminton, track and field, you name it, get nervous. But here is the difference: It's how these world-class performers manage and control their nerves. They view the energy as positive and reap the benefits of empowering self-talk and happy thoughts.

International Hall of Famer and winner of 39 grand slam titles Billie Jean King described pressure as a privilege. She said, "Pressure is a privilege as it only comes to them who truly earn it." In fact, it just so happens to be the title of her book.

Winners know that pressure makes them better. Whether you are a golfer or a tennis player, a Fortune 500 CEO, an actor, or a parent, the way you view that energy will determine how you deal with all kinds of pressure. Those with a winner's attitude and mindset embrace the challenge. You can talk yourself into, or out of, almost anything. Those with a winner's attitude and mindset view their outlook on things as their greatest weapon.

When others don't think something's possible, winners consistently see it as a great opportunity to succeed and make the impossible, possible. You can, too. Instead of saying, "Why me?" people with a winner's attitude and mindset say, "Try me!"

Harness your energy in a positive way
when adversity and challenges arise.
When you do this,
you develop grit and resilience –
two things that provide you
with a distinct competitive advantage.

Chapter 22

Finding Joy Is a Choice

I believe that to live a rich and abundant life, you must make true joy and happiness a conscious choice. No matter how much money or fame, no matter how many trophies, investments, or material things you may possess, in the end they cannot fulfill you if you aren't happy within yourself. Outward success without inner happiness and fulfillment is, in my opinion, only failure in the end.

A few years ago I realized that two beliefs were holding me back from experiencing real joy. The first was that I had the "never good enough" mentality that I mentioned earlier. The second was a trust problem. Having been let down in a few relationships, both personal and professional, I found it hard to trust others. It has been said that you will be hurt occasionally if you trust too much, but as I've experienced, you won't find true joy if you don't trust enough.

A quality I've discovered in some of the happiest and most joyful people in the world is that they don't attach themselves to things that can be taken away in an instant. Some of the most joyful people have absolutely nothing. Having traveled to such places as the poverty slums of South Africa and Thailand, I have witnessed happier and more joyful people there than I have in some of the wealthiest zip codes in the United States of America – Beverly Hills to Palm Beach. Sometimes people who are worth more money than they can spend, I've discovered, are unhappy because they have fallen victim to the "want more" mentality and focus on comparing, criticizing and judging others.

It's funny, but when I ask people what they want in life, the first thing they say is happiness. My follow-up question usually asks what is holding them back from being happy and joyful. The answers usually range from "I don't know really" to "I suppose when I get that promotion" to "when I win that tournament or championship." They are thinking that when they reach a milestone or achieve something, that happiness will appear. Truth is, it might come, but it lasts for only a very short time. It's a bit like buying a new car or a new pair of shoes; it might make you happy for a few days or weeks, but after a while, things simply become just like all the other achievements or materials you possess, and the want-more mentality kicks in. I've even spent time with Olympic gold medalists and people who've made multiple millions of dollars thinking those things would bring them certain happiness. But *stuff* just doesn't do it.

Regardless of your past circumstances or current situation, you get to choose if you will be happy or not. You see, joy and happiness are not a destination, but rather a choice. Happiness doesn't come to you; you go to it. Greatness is about celebrating life, and I believe that it can't be achieved without being grateful and appreciative of the little things you have in your life.

Sitting in a waiting lounge in the Atlanta airport one evening, I listened to an interview with Philadelphia Eagles Super Bowl champion quarterback Nick Foles. Prior to the Eagles winning the 2018 Super Bowl and after some frustrating seasons, Foles realized he was placing an enormous amount of pressure on himself; he was no longer enjoying the game. It was only after changing his outlook and mindset, realizing the joy in what he was doing and focusing on gratitude and love that he was able to find more fulfillment and achieve his best performances.

The way to joy and happiness, as I mentioned earlier, is in essence through the relationship you have with yourself. If you can't have a meaningful and healthy relationship with yourself, you can't have a healthy relationship with the world. It does indeed start inside. If you feel you are unworthy, are continually beating yourself up over the past or are blaming yourself for your past mistakes, you will never allow yourself to experience joy and feel the freedom to live the life you were meant to have. You have to first let go of the past in order to move forward into the future. You can't discover new destinations without leaving the shore.

Don't put the key to your happiness in someone else's pocket. Your passion evaporates when you say yes to things that you don't care about. Minimize doing anything that you don't feel passionate about and do so unapologetically, though respectfully.

Don't let society tell you what it means to be happy either. That is for you alone to work out. Don't ever feel the need to prove yourself to anyone to be liked or appreciated. Being accepted by others when you don't accept yourself is just an illusion. Real happiness and joy come from accepting yourself and being authentic with your intentions. If that isn't good enough for certain people in your life, perhaps they aren't good enough to be in your life.

10 Ways to Increase Your Joy and Happiness

1. Be grateful
2. Give of your time, and help others
3. Appreciate the small things in life more
4. Enjoy the company of those you love
5. Be more accepting of yourself

6.   Watch your favorite show or a great comedy

7.   Improve your self-talk

8.   Do more of the things you love to do

9.   Take care of your health

10. Do not take yourself so seriously

Make a commitment right now to be more joyful every day. Find the smallest things and focus on gratitude and love. What are you waiting for?

Remember that life doesn't have to be
perfect for you to find joy and happiness.
It's a choice and
it begins with the mindset you choose,
regardless of your circumstances.

Chapter 23

Upgrade Your Mindset

Upgrade your attitude and mindset, and you will upgrade your life. Free yourself from limiting thoughts. Unlearn the ideas that are holding you back. Seek to empower yourself and build a future on the foundations of faith and optimism.

Do you have faith in yourself? Do you contemplate your day, week, life with optimism? The answers to these questions have an enormous impact on your life. For starters, they affect your attitude, your energy, your body language, your mood, your personality and more. They are not just a game changer; they define the rules of your game. Speak to yourself with only those words that build you up, and none of those that break you down. Bring more positivity into your life. Delete the negativity. What are you saying to keep yourself ahead in the point count?

Being positive doesn't mean you don't face moments of negativity and doubt. People with winning attitudes and positive outlooks also face damaging thoughts. The main difference, however, lies in how quickly positive people get rid of them. Through deliberate practice over weeks, months and years, they have trained their minds to quickly eliminate destructive ideas and replace them with positive and self-empowering ones.

It happens to me, too. Each day I'm attacked by negative thoughts, but I don't entertain them. I eradicate them quickly and substitute constructive ones. It does take time to develop.

People from many different walks of life come to me for help with developing their mindsets. They want to become more positive, more mentally tough and stronger. From the beginning I explain that changing oneself into a more positive person is harder than they think. This is not to discourage them, but to remind them that where they are today is the result of beliefs, thoughts and behaviors formed over a lifetime. Changing your mindset is much like learning a new language! To develop a more positive and optimistic outlook, you have to reprogram the brain, set new beliefs, and learn to speak in a winners-like language. Instead of focusing on how things are, focus your energy on how you want things to be. Create a mental picture of it. This is the only way to bring about a progressive and positive change in your life.

Each day you are faced with a choice. Either you keep yourself back and limit your incredible potential by hanging onto self-defeating thoughts and self-defeating beliefs, or each day you choose to get up, feel grateful and get out there and make your mental picture a reality.

If you were to rate what you say to yourself on a scale of 1 to 10, what score would you give yourself? If it's less than an 8, then you are holding yourself back from your greatest potential. You are robbing yourself of self-confidence and self-belief. It comes back to one of my favorite (and one of the most basic) truths, that self-belief is an inside-out job. What you repeat day after day, year after year will manifest in your life. Positive thoughts, positive life. The opposite is true as well. Many years back when I was living in South Africa, I heard the late great Nelson Mandela speak one of my favorite quotes:

> Our deepest fear is not that we are inadequate. Our deepest fear is that we are powerful beyond measure. It is our light, not our darkness that most

frightens us. We ask ourselves, "Who am I to be brilliant, gorgeous, talented, fabulous?" Actually, who are you not to be? Your playing small does not serve the world. There is nothing enlightened about shrinking so that other people won't feel insecure around you. We are all meant to shine, as children do. It's not just in some of us; it's in everyone. And as we let our own light shine, we unconsciously give other people permission to do the same. As we are liberated from our own fear, our presence automatically liberates others.

I love that Nelson Mandela says, "It's not just in some of us; it's in everyone." This includes you. Why wait for tomorrow to make that change? Do it today; in fact, make that decision right now. Our greatest life lies ahead of us – isn't that exciting? No matter what has happened in the past, it is in the past. Once you upgrade your mindset, once you replace negative thoughts with positives ones, you will start having a more positive and abundant life.

If you want good things in life, you have to step out of your comfort zone, believe in yourself, and pursue your goals and dreams with passion every day.

———————————————

Once your mindset changes, everything else changes, too. Focus on all the good things happening in your life right now, and look forward to the good things that will be coming in the future.

SECTION 4

SELF-DISCIPLINE

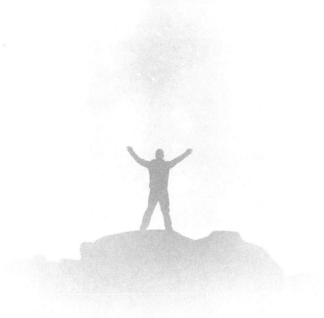

Chapter 24

Self-discipline Is Foundational to All Success

No one lazy or unmotivated makes it to the top. Achieving anything of significance demands a high level of self-discipline and habits geared toward excellence. Be it reaching a high level in sports or climbing the corporate ladder, you will need dedication and a deep desire to work hard. When one combines self-discipline with a winning attitude, excellence occurs.

"What exactly is self-discipline?" you ask. Well, any group of people will probably give you an assortment of different answers. Through the experiences of my own life and observing others, I've discovered that discipline is one of the most important attributes in creating the lifestyle you want and giving you the freedom to do what it is you wish to do. I have always believed that success lies in doing what others don't like to do or won't do. It lies in going to where others aren't willing to go. When you are willing to do the things that others aren't willing to do, opportunities arise and doors open.

One thing for sure is that the more self-discipline you have, the more freedom it eventually makes possible in your life. The same principle applies to greatness – the more self-discipline you have, the more greatness, in whatever area of life, you will eventually achieve. Personally, I believe discipline gives you the chance to design the life you wish to lead – I call it living by design. I know that the 80-hour work weeks I put in in the first half of my career, doing the things that others didn't want to do, or going to where others didn't like to go, gave me the freedom I have today. I now get to choose what my day looks like. I now work the hours I want. I now have the freedom to work and collaborate with the people I want to. The years of discipline have now given me the freedom to choose. Today, I'm blessed to wake up and decide how my day will be, but it wouldn't have been this way without the foundations of years and years of self-discipline and hard work.

Let's get clear about what self-discipline is and isn't:

- Self-discipline is not punishment like some think it is. It's a skill that's needed in order to achieve greatness and more favorable outcomes.

- Self-discipline is not something you are born with. Like a winning attitude, it's something you get to choose each day.

- The more self-discipline you have the more freedom you'll eventually have (credit: Jocko Willink).

- Self-discipline is what the champions and high performers have more of than even their fellow achievers.

Jocko Willink, the decorated retired Navy SEAL officer and author of the book *Extreme Ownership* said it best:

Freedom is what everyone wants – to be able to act and live with freedom. But the only way to get to a place of freedom is through discipline. If you want more financial freedom, you have to have financial discipline. If you want more free time, you have to follow a more disciplined time management system. If you want more, you also have to have the discipline to say no to things that eat up your time with no payback – things like random YouTube videos, click-bait on the internet, and even events that you agree to attend when you know you won't want to be there. *Discipline = freedom* applies to every aspect of life: If you want more freedom, get more discipline.

From a very young age I wanted to be a champion. It didn't really matter what sport. I simply wanted to be a champion. I was probably around the age of 10 when I set out on this journey. I might not have realized it at the time, but I was not your regular 10-year-old kid. I could spend hours running, biking and playing any sport that came my way. In fact, in school, I participated in eight sports! I eventually went on to represent my country, South Africa, five times in the world championships in the sport of duathlon (running and cycling). One year I ran 12 marathons, and the next year I ran 7 marathons and 7 half marathons in 7 weeks. Looking back, I see that some of my training routines were ruthless. Come rain, snow or heat, I'd be out doing more than anyone else. My motivation was always to never be outworked. I was so disciplined that I decided as a teenager that I would never let a drop of alcohol touch my lips until I'd finished my professional career, a pledge I stood by until I did my last race at the age of 33. I was so disciplined I didn't have fast food for 12 years. A dessert might be a vanilla protein shake. I trained Christmas Day, New Year's morning – it didn't matter what time or day it was! I believe it was from these early days in my life that I was able to build a high level of self-discipline, a decision that has served me well in many areas in my life to this day.

I am sometimes asked, "How does one acquire more self-discipline?" I believe self-discipline comes from your greater reason for doing something, your "why." When your why, your purpose, is great, your desire to be committed and your level of discipline will be heightened. I always like to go back to the example of when people set New Year's resolutions, and why the vast majority fail come February. It's because their purpose wasn't strong enough. It was more superficial than internal.

The ultimate competitive advantage is the ability to discipline your mind to create the energy required for the action you need. Every time you see a champion or individual succeed, you can be very sure that you're looking at someone who has paid great attention to the details of self-discipline, worked extremely hard and acquired a winning attitude and mindset.

Use consistent self-discipline now
so you can enjoy the freedom
to live the life you want in the future.

Chapter 25

A Winner's Attitude Involves Daily Investment

W ould you like to know one of the most important reasons that some people succeed and others do not? The ones who succeed invest in themselves daily. They invest in their relationships, in their career, and in their health (among many other vital areas) on a daily basis. Despite obstacles and challenges, these people are the winners in life because they have decided to be. They are the ones who have adopted an attitude of "if it's meant to be, it's up to me." They are the more action and less talk kind of people.

Two such people? One was a fellow speaker at a conference in New York who referred to a simple adage that has stuck with me. He said, "Those who invest go further than the rest." Amazing how some simple quotes just stick with you, right? The other was someone who knows quite well where best to place your resources. Business magnate, billionaire investor and philanthropist Warren Buffet advised, "The most important investment you can make is in yourself."

One of the key elements in developing a winning attitude and mindset is that you have to be intentional and strategic about investing in yourself. What do I mean by this? You need to intentionally set aside time each day to invest in the most important facets of life. I live by a personal motto that goes "live each day like you are running out of time." The truth is, we are. When I put my head on the pillow at night, I want to know I did all I could today in order to live out my greater purpose and vision.

In my book *Champion Minded* I talk about the "15-90." If you spend just 15 minutes per day investing in a particular area, be it on bettering a skill, practicing an instrument or learning a new language, those 15 minutes per day will add up to over 90 hours per year. Think about the fact that champions do extra. Those extra minutes they put in make the difference in the end.

The hours add up quickly. An extra

15 minutes a day = 91.25 hours a year

30 minutes a day = 182.5 hours a year

45 minutes a day = 271.75 hours a year

60 minutes a day = 365 hours a year

When you spend time on yourself growing and making progress, be it in life, relationships, career, etc., you become fulfilled. And when you feel fulfilled, you more easily develop a winning attitude. People who are aiming for greatness don't find the time; they make it. They don't use the old "I don't have time" excuse. All that means is that self-improvement is not important enough to them. If you are on Facebook or social media just scrolling, then you have time. You simply made a different choice. If something means enough to you, you will have the time, period.

People who are aiming for greatness don't get sidetracked and distracted from what needs to be done in order to progress. Each day they invest in their health, their relationships, their career, their spiritual side, and other important areas of their lives. They plan for it. They don't let other things get in the way. Recently I attended a Leaders Evening in Manchester, England, where Siemens UK CEO Jurgen Maier was the invited speaker. He emphasized, "Never stop upgrading and investing in yourself."

Remember that investing even a few minutes per day in important areas of your life is better than doing nothing and that it will be one of the best returns on investment you can get. Whether it's time spent learning a new skill, developing yourself personally or professionally, tapping into your creativity or hiring a coach, investing in yourself is one of the major keys to realizing and achieving your greatness.

9 Ways to Invest in Yourself

1. Read more
2. Exercise – hire a trainer
3. Listen to podcasts
4. Watch interesting documentaries, TED talks or educational programs
5. Go to workshops/seminars
6. Study or enroll in a new course
7. Speak to different people in different sectors and industries
8. Take someone you can learn from out for coffee or lunch
9. Find a mentor/coach in the area you want to get better at

---

*The height of your success is
in direct proportion to the level
of your personal development.
People with winning attitudes and mindsets
invest in themselves daily.*

Chapter 26

A Winning Attitude
Is About Giving the Extra 5%

I'll admit that I was never really that great a student, and although I wasn't bad at sports, I was never the first choice on a team or in PE class. However, one thing I knew from a young age was that if I worked harder than anyone else and had a great attitude, I could achieve great things. In fact, this knowledge was one of the main reasons I wrote Champion Minded – to inspire those with less academic inclination or raw talent to know that they can still achieve great things if they apply themselves. I knew that I had achieved things beyond what most of my coaches thought possible when I was younger, so why not keep the ball rolling?

I have two 5% rules. One, which we'll look at in Chapter 30, is that a major reason why the top 5% of successful people are at the top – whether in business, sports or academia – is that they are willing to do more than what is asked of them. My other 5% rule is that by consistently giving an extra 5% of effort, you can succeed beyond any predictions. I knew from a young age that going the extra mile was where I would be able to get my edge. As I went along in life, I was fueled by seeing my progress from just doing that extra 5% more than anyone else.

I made sure I was first at practice and last to leave in order to better my skills. It worked. My first big success was that I become a national junior champion in Duathlon (running and biking) as well as going on to successfully compete in five world championships over a span of nine years.

I always knew that I would get my advantage from outworking others, especially those who were more talented or skilled than I was. You could say that I got a kick out of it. I know in my heart that if I had done only as much as my teammates or what my coaches had of asked from me, I wouldn't have achieved what I did. In fact, I still live by the give 5% more rule in all I do. Becoming successful isn't rocket science. It's putting in the work every day and keeping a great attitude.

Today, when I speak to large groups and especially young students in colleges around the United States, I love to talk about willingly doing what others don't feel like doing. It gives you more opportunities in life. You see, when you are willing to consistently and continually go that extra 5%, you make it hard for decision makers to not to want to select you, recruit you, hire you, contract you or promote you. When you go the extra mile, especially with a winning attitude, you will begin to attract endless opportunities and start to see doors opening right in front of you.

In a sports team setting, coaches have two reasons for wanting a player who consistently gives the extra 5%. Of course they will have one spectacularly hard worker. The bonus is that that one hard worker inspires others to follow the example.

One great example of going the extra mile is former Olympic gymnast and gold medalist Peter Vidmar. Peter realized that if he worked just 15 minutes extra a day after normal practice time (which I mentioned earlier), that would add up to an extra 90 hours a year. Did it make a difference? You bet it did! He went on to win the gold medal in the men's pommel horse event by the slightest of margins in the 1984 Los Angeles Olympics. Peter understood the extra 5% effect.

Truth is, I've never met a coach, boss, manager, leader or teacher who didn't love an athlete, employee, student who did the extra work to make things happen. A winning attitude will eventually reward you. Don't expect it overnight; like Peter, keep working on it consistently, and over time you will reap the benefits.

The only person who can decide whether your future will be what you are dreaming of or just a dream of what might have been is you. Becoming successful isn't rocket science. It's about putting in the extra 5% every day. Do it, and do it with a smile.

Imagine the difference in your outcomes
if you were to give an extra 5% more effort.

Chapter 27

Learn to Say No
When It's Necessary

I'll admit that until a few years ago, I struggled with saying no to people who asked me for something. Since then I've learned that developing a winning attitude and mindset requires that you have to be 100% honest with yourself and be firm with others. You have only so much energy, and you have to be careful where that energy goes. I've learned that saying yes to things I didn't want to do, and really didn't need to do, only made me unhappy and stole my passion. Don't get me wrong, I absolutely love to serve and help people, but there are times when a person simply has to say no.

Do you sometimes wish you could just do this – put your foot down and say no, especially without feeling guilty about it? Many of us feel compelled to agree to every request, and would rather juggle a ton of projects than refuse to help, even if we are left with no time for ourselves. We don't want to hurt anyone's feelings or let anyone down. When you are in this kind of mindset, the one who loses most of the time is you.

It is important to set your boundaries. Others need to know them, and it is your responsibility to set them. Maybe it's time to say goodbye to being a people pleaser or trying to be the fixer of every problem and learn how to confidently say no without feeling bad about it.

I used to say yes to every request, be it helping unpack boxes, taking on one more client or taking another speaking engagement. The result eventually was that my quality and attention to details began to waiver as my energy and enthusiasm became depleted. And when I got back home, my energy and presence for those closest to me, my friends and family, would be on empty. The result was that they would not be getting the best of me. I've learned the importance of valuing my own time and energy, and I no longer feel selfish about it. If I don't take care of myself first, then how can I take care of those around me who matter most?

After my first book, *7 Keys to Being a Great Coach*, was released, I was getting over 100 emails a week related to the book. At the end of many long days I found myself returning to my office or hotel room and trying to reply to them all. It was crazy, and some days ended at 2 a.m.! I needed to reevaluate my schedule and how valuable my time and energy are. Also, it was important for me to remember my priorities and not let other things get in the way.

When traveling I often get asked to dinner, and I sometimes have to respectfully decline. I need to stick to my priorities, which are first and foremost my health, energy and responsibilities. Saying yes to every request and being out until late at dinners deplete my energy for the next day and days after that. That doesn't mean I always turn down these dinners or functions; in fact, they are very enjoyable and an important way to build relationships and connections, but I usually excuse myself early if I do attend. I have to prioritize the next morning and how I start my day. It sets up the rest of the day.

I would say that the biggest difference between the first half of my career and now is that in the beginning I said yes to everything. These days, now more established and having been able to design the life I want (living by design), I am able to say no more often, which is a privilege. I believe that the first 10-15 years of your career are the building phases as that is where all the groundwork is laid. It is a time when, even though you still have to decide what does need and what does not need to be done, you still have to say yes more often in order to lay your foundation. You do have to put in those years and years of grind and time and prove your credibility. However, once you become more established and in demand for what you do, you begin to have the luxury of choosing your projects and work.

Learning to say no is one of the most effective ways to increase your focus and overall productivity. Saying no will help you better invest time and energy into things that produce better results. Saying no to the things that don't matter or matter less allows you to say yes to the things that really do matter. It's not always easy, I know, but learning to say no can earn you respect from yourself as well as from those around you.

Learning how and when to say no helps you to

1. free up more time to do the things you want to do or need to do

2. choose what does and what doesn't fit with your greater vision and purpose

3. realize what you simply don't enjoy doing anymore

4. face the fact that with some people it's always a take-take. It's important to say no to people who don't support you, people who might manipulate you, people who are always in some way using you. Making this decision also helps you find the win-win relationships that boost your quality of life. Those people who are always taking eventually drain your soul and make you feel bad.

5. notice what is colliding with more important things in your life, like family commitments and other priorities

3 Ways to Effectively Say No

1. Step up and just say it.

Stop worrying what the other person will think. Don't beat around the bush or offer excuses about why you can't or won't. This only provides an opening for the other person. Provide a brief explanation if you feel you really need to; however, don't feel compelled to. The less said the better.

2. Be firm and be selfish in the appropriate way.

First, if someone can't accept your no, then you know the person is probably not a true friend or doesn't respect you and your time. Stand firm, and don't feel compelled to give in just because that person is uncomfortable. Second, be selfish in the appropriate way. It is, after all, your time. If you don't put your needs first, then you will always be unhappy.

3. Set boundaries.

People need to know where they stand. They need to know where your boundaries are and what your standards are. If you don't let them know, then they will keep testing them. When you are definite about your boundaries, others will stop push-push-pushing you.

It's not always selfish to put yourself first.
When you truly understand
the dynamic and your role,
you won't feel worried about the consequences
of sometimes having to say no to others.

Chapter 28

Winners Are Never Outworked

Hard work pays off. Maybe not always when you want it to, but eventually it does. Comedian Kevin Hart once said, "Everybody wants to be famous, but nobody wants to do the work. I live by that. You grind hard so you can play hard. At the end of the day, you put in all the work, and eventually it will pay off. It could be in a year, it could be in 10 years. Eventually, your hard work will pay off." If talent were primary, the best people would always win. If strategy were primary, the best plan would always win. But that's not what happens. Not in business, not in sports and not in life. However, one thing I know is that opportunity always lies on the other side of hard work. You won't achieve anything by simply wishing for it. It doesn't work that way. You've got to get out there, hustle and work your butt off every single day.

From an early age I knew I wasn't the most talented or skilled. Two of my worst classes were English and biology. Little did I know that many years later they would become the two most important subjects in my career – writing and understanding the human body. See how purpose can propel you to places you never thought you could go?

When I think back, I realize that I'm grateful that I struggled through my younger years. It gave me an incentive and reason to train harder. I didn't mind winning or losing. As long as I knew I gave it my all, that was good enough for me. Defeat or rejection gave me another reason to do better. I'm not going to lie – it wasn't exactly pleasurable at times, but what it taught me was a deep level of grit, resilience and determination, qualities that take you much further in life than just game skills or an impressive report card.

My message is this: An A on that report card is great, but an A in life – Attitude – trumps everything. You might be outsmarted by people more brilliant than you, out-sprinted by people who are faster than you, outmaneuvered by people more connected than you, but if you refuse to be outworked, you're almost guaranteed to be successful in the area you have chosen to pursue, and live a life of greatness.

Often I come across people who say they "want it bad," but their actions don't show it. Talk is cheap. Your effort level will always prove your intensions. If you want it bad enough, you will do what it takes. No excuses. No complaining. No blaming. New York Yankees legend Derek Jeter said it best: "There may be people who have more talent than you, but there's no excuse for anyone to work harder than you do – and I believe that."

Those with a winning attitude and mindset just simply refuse to be outworked. To outwork others, you've got to be willing to get uncomfortable – in fact very uncomfortable. I'm talking early and late, places you don't want to go and things you don't want to do, plus putting up with pain. Learn to love the hard problems. And do the hard stuff first, because if you don't, it won't get done.

One day, all those late nights and early mornings will pay off. Rising to the top involves never allowing yourself to be outworked. Keep going. Keep hustling. Trust me, all that effort will be worth it in the end. Win or lose, at least you will have no regrets.

To achieve the shine,
you need to embrace the grind!

Chapter 29

Winning Habits
Determine Your Destiny

I believe that the level of your self-discipline is revealed by the lifestyle you lead and the habits you keep. Aristotle said, "We become what we repeatedly do. Excellence is not an act; it's a habit." In other words, we become our habits; we are the sum of our habits. When we allow bad habits to take over, they dramatically impede our path to success. The challenge that we face is that bad habits are insidious, creeping up on us slowly until we don't even notice the damage they're causing. Think about that chocolate after dinner every night or those cookies with every cup of tea or coffee.

When it comes to habits, one of the big myths is the belief that it takes 21 days for a good habit to form. I don't believe this for a moment. In my experience it takes at least 90 days to build a solid habit and only 9 days to lose it. I call it the 90/9 rule. The longer you practice a good habit, the more ingrained it becomes. Be consistent.

The fastest way to achieve your potential and your goals is through your level of commitment. When you are fully committed to something, nothing else will stand in your way – unless, of course, you have bad habits. Yet if your purpose and commitment are strong enough, you can break those bad habits.

The level of your success comes down to the level of self-discipline you have in your daily habits – getting rid of the bad ones and being steadfast with the good ones. Set high standards for yourself and focus on the positive daily behaviors that support them. Your self-discipline with these behaviors creates the winning habits that determine how much freedom and choice you get to have in life.

Here are 5 ways to ensure good habits:

1. Start small.

One of the biggest mistakes people make when they want to make changes in their life or career is to take on too much. For example, they want to lose weight and get in shape, so they radically change their diet and plan to go to the gym seven days a week, only to totally bomb out a few days or weeks later. Why is this? The unrealistic goals they have set for themselves are overwhelming. The right approach is to start small. Set a more reasonable goal like getting to the gym three times a week to start with. Understand that every big habit is supported by many smaller habits and decisions. Find the small habit and develop that one first, and change one at a time.

2. Build routines.

The most successful people I've studied all have this in common – they have daily routines. Waking up and knowing the game plan for your day is essential. If you are planning to get in shape, for example, set a specific time to go to the gym and stick to it no matter what. The day goes better for me if I do it first thing in the morning so I have more control of my day and other things don't get in the way. So, for example, if I have to travel, I get started extra early. Find out what works best for you.

3. *See* it as much as possible!

Know exactly what you want. Get clear on who you are and what you want to become by writing it down. See it every day. When I have wanted to develop a new habit, I have even used sticky notes as reminders. For example, I wanted to develop the habit of drinking more water, so I left water bottles around the house, on my office desk, in the car, in my bags, etc. When you see it more and make it visual, it will better remind you what to do.

4. Journal your progress.

There is no better feeling than achieving your daily goals. The secret is not to wait for only the big ones. Celebrate your daily ones – all those little victories you have in a day. Each evening I like to write a few down and self-reflect. Actually seeing what I've accomplished helps me stay motivated and on track. Without proper reflection, the habits don't have proper meaning. By applying your own meaning, you can accelerate your progress. Positive reinforcement will fuel additional motivation and achievement.

5. Have people around to remind you.

Surround yourself only with people who are going to lift you higher. Have them hold you accountable with reminders. Don't look for the yes people, those who tell you only what you want to hear. The right people will make sure you are on track and do it in a positive way. I do this when I set a big goal like running a marathon. I tell those closest to me and they keep me accountable. This kind of supporter will give you that kick in the butt when needed.

Last but not least, habits help you do things consistently, without having to think about the entire process all the time. Those with a winning attitude and mindset have developed great habits over time – habits that take them to where they want to go. Remember that the choices you make today form your habits of tomorrow. Success is a result of staying consistent in the good daily habits.

_____

Your beliefs become your thoughts,
Your thoughts become your words,
Your words become your actions,
Your actions become your habits,
Your habits become your values,
Your values become your destiny.

– Mahatma Gandhi

Chapter 30

Winners Do More

If you want to succeed in life, then be the person who does more than what's been asked of them. As I mentioned earlier, I have two 5% rules. The one we discussed in Chapter 26 is that by consistently giving an extra 5% of effort, you can succeed beyond any predictions. The other is that a major reason the top 5% of successful people reach the top, in whatever area, is that they are willing to do more than what is asked of them – more than the other 95%.

Achieving significance in what you are pursuing requires meeting more than basic expectations. If you want to be average, that's fine; then just do just enough or just what's been asked. Finding your greatness and rising to the top involve being willing to go the extra mile. They require a commitment to persistence and excellence.

You might have more experience or have a higher degree than the next person, but if they have a winning attitude and better work ethic, don't be surprised if they leapfrog you on the way. Success and happiness don't come to you, you go to them. When Golden State Warriors head coach Steve Kerr was asked recently what made his team so successful, he put it down to their attitude and the work ethic within their culture. He said that players like Steph Curry and Klay Thompson usually stay after regular practice to spend an extra 45 minutes to an hour working on their skills. Kerr put their success down to the players wanting to, and being willing to, do more.

Another great example of a do-more mentality was the Mamba, Kobe Bryant. His work ethic was off the charts, too. Kobe was known to be in the gym at 4:30 a.m., long before the rest of his teammates arrived at the facility. Herein lies the reason these players stood out above their world-class teammates and opponents. True champions do more. They don't need to be asked. They believe in the extra work. They believe that all the little bits of extra effort will eventually pay off.

In my athletic career, it wasn't by doing just enough that I became a world-class athlete who competed in five world championships and, after that, got to work with some of the finest athletes on planet earth. I had to do more – much more. When others were partying or taking days off, I was working my butt off, double time. It was 4:00 a.m. mornings and into bed at 11:00 p.m. I worked two part-time jobs a day while balancing four to five hours training a day. When training and competing, I'd be on the road sleeping in garages, in attics, on people's couches, and sometimes in train stations – all in pursuit of my athletic goals. I didn't mind because I was willing to do what it took to reach them. I built some serious grit and resilience in those days. These days I hear athletes complaining about staying in a three- or four-star hotel or about the food provided for them at the tournaments – I would have given my left hand for those luxuries.

That's why I always go back to my 5% theory. Those who achieve greatness are willing to go where others won't go and do what others won't to do. In my experience, the ones who get ahead and realize their potential had this exact mindset – a winning one. They had what I call in my book Champion Minded the one-more mentality, doing that one extra rep in the gym when your muscles are screaming at you to stop, that one extra set of hill sprints in the pouring rain when the rest of your team has gone home or that one extra project at the office that no one else wants to do. People who succeed do it because they know that hard work pays off. They do it because it's their journey.

Success comes at a price. It involves early mornings and late nights. When writing my books, I had to commit to getting up earlier and going to bed later. I even got rid of my TV. When people ask how I found the time among all my other commitments to write three books in three years, I tell them exactly that – get rid of distractions! I had lots of traveling, speaking, meetings and exercise, but I wrote on planes and trains and in airports and hotel rooms. This, I believe, is the main difference between those who are not willing to go the extra distance or put in the hours and those who regularly achieve their goals. It comes down to discipline and consistency.

The great thing about doing the extra work is that it requires no special talent or skills. It simply requires a choice of attitude and mindset, something available to every single one of us. So, you want to be great? You want to be successful? Well, what are you willing to do to get there? And, even more importantly, what are you willing to give up to get there?

Here's the cool thing about the extra mile: There are no crowds lining the extra mile, no spectators, no lights, no cameras, nothing. Just you and the empty road. On one hand, it's the hardest mile you will ever travel, but it's the only path that will lead to lasting success in life. On the other hand, the harder you work the less competition you have. The legendary soccer player and World Cup winner Mia Hamm said, "The vision of a champion is bent over, drenched in sweat, at the point of exhaustion, when nobody else is looking."

The top 5% of successful people, be it in career or in life, are consistently willing to do more, to give more, to be more.

A major reason why the top 5% succeed,
be it in sports, business or any other field,
is this:
They are willing to do
more than what's been asked of them.

SECTION 5

ROLE MODELS

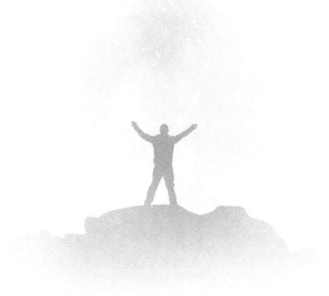

Chapter 31

Paul Serves More than Just Coffee

It was on my connection flying back home from Dallas to Fort Lauderdale that I had a layover in Atlanta. I had an hour and a half till my next flight, so I headed to the Starbucks to grab a cup of coffee. As I approached, I noticed there was a queue of 12-15 people. No problem, I thought. I had enough time.

Then I noticed that there was only one person working behind the counter, a gentleman probably in his mid-twenties. Usually in a busy airport like Hartsfield Jackson, you expect to see at least three or four baristas at a Starbucks, but on this occasion, it was only Paul (according to his name badge).

Who knows why he was all alone? What struck me first was that instead of looking stressed (like most people in this situation), Paul looked relaxed and as cool as a cucumber. Taking the orders, making coffees, warming up sandwiches, taking payments – Paul was doing it all. Not only was he running the show like a pro, but at the same time, he chatted casually with his customers. All this in between his humming and singing while he performed three people's jobs at once.

I saw immediately that Paul had a winner's attitude. In fact, he was the kind of guy I'd hire in a heartbeat. Even if he were skilled only to make and serve and coffee, I'd hire his attitude over skills, because skills can be taught.

Usually in a situation like this, it wouldn't be uncommon to find a few irritated and impatient customers in line. But of all the people in the long line in front of me and behind me, no one seemed annoyed. How could this be? Well, it was simple. Through Paul's attitude and ability to understand what was in his control (and what wasn't), he was able to create a relaxed and pleasant environment.

Now, you would probably agree that Paul had every right to feel annoyed, angry and upset over the situation, but his attitude changed not only his own experience, but that of each of his customers as well. Paul set the tone.

It was probably 25 minutes before I got to the front of the line. Paul greeted me with a smile that could easily appear in a Colgate ad. As with the other customers, he asked how my day had been and where I was flying to. After answering him, I immediately complimented him on how he was handling things and told him how incredibly impressed I was. I asked him what his secret was to handling such a situation, and what he told me I'll probably never forget. He said, "I get to choose my attitude. I can be disgruntled by the situation of being alone here at the moment, or I can choose to keep a positive attitude and enjoy my work. I also completely understand how these people feel. Some have been flying for hours and are exhausted and all they want is a nice cup of coffee. So the way I see it is that I am the one who gets to give them that coffee. I get to put a smile on their faces and wish them safe travels to wherever they may be going to next." Wow! I was blown away. Talk about a winning attitude and someone who understands what real empathy means!

Now there are a few lessons to be learned here. First, Paul was able to influence the environment he was in by being calm, relaxed and happy. Second, through his attitude and efforts, the people who were waiting appreciated how he was handling things. Last but not least, walking away from that Starbucks, I felt reenergized from spending just a few minutes around someone with a contagious, winning attitude. Truth be told, because I had enough time until my next flight, I sat down at the opposite gate and enjoyed this exhibition of a winning attitude and mindset.

You get to choose how you respond to adverse situations. You can choose to be grumpy, irritated or angry, or you can be like Paul and choose to make the experience a better one, even when just serving coffee.

Always aim to be the type of energy that,
no matter where you go,
you add value to the spaces and
lives of those around you.

Chapter 32

Attitude Is a Choice

They say that the real test and proof of a man's character and resilience is when adversity hits. In 2018, a year after his diagnosis, my very dear friend Oliver Stephens lost his battle with histiocytosis, a rare form of cancer. Ollie made a difference to every person he came into contact with and got way more out of his life than people even twice his age.

Ollie was an amazing tennis coach who had dreams of going to the very top. He was passionate about what he did and was incredibly invested in his personal growth. He was part of my "buddies' book club" where several friends share books and ideas. He was one of the funniest and most compassionate individuals I ever knew. Ollie was also a wonderful husband to Milena; in fact, they had gotten married just two years earlier. Starting in April 2016 Ollie spent his last year at the University of Miami hospital, going home only once to see his beloved dog, Emma, who he missed dearly. Ollie was only 42 when he left us.

Each week, I made the drive down to Miami from Boca Raton, always eager to visit my good friend, someone who always brightened the day of everyone he came into contact with. Even on his toughest days, when he got pierced by needle after needle, he was still able to laugh and joke with the nurses, his wife and anyone who was nearby. His attitude was incredible. Everyone loved Ollie's sense of humor and energy – they were contagious. When you were with him, you couldn't help but feel happy.

Ollie was such a source of comfort and inspiration for me that sometimes I'd sit bedside and share my worries and concerns. Later on, even on his darkest days when he was so weak that he couldn't lift his hand or even open eyes, he was still able to mumble to me, "Allistair, attitude is a choice." In fact, these four words were Ollie's personal motto. I even have a photo of his two clenched fists with the letters A-T-T-I-T-U-D-E displayed on the base bones of his eight fingers.

It's easy to have a winning attitude when everything is going well, but how is it when adversity strikes? When I complain or am acting negatively, my mind still reverts to those four words: Attitude is a choice. Knowing what Ollie went through puts things into perspective for me when I am feeling sorry for myself or not being grateful. It gets my attitude back on track.

Whatever your circumstances, attitude comes down to a choice; you can choose whether to let external things affect it or not. The legacy Ollie left is about choosing a positive mental attitude. He walked his talk. RIP, my good friend. I miss you.

Attitude is a choice.

– Ollie Stephens

Chapter 33

Elevating Others Elevates You

After being away for three weeks on an overseas work trip, one of my first stops on the way home was to pick up groceries at my local supermarket. I love this place because they usually hire senior citizens and people with disabilities, and support various charities and organizations. On this particular day, my bag packer Jose was chatting enthusiastically with the cashier. During his dialogue with her, he was packing customers' bags, humming and singing to himself and smiling. Instantly I felt a great energy around him.

After wishing the customer before me a great day and weekend, he fixed his eyes on me and said, "Good day, young man. Looks like you certainly keep fit!" I said, "Thank you" and smiled. As he was packing my groceries into the bags, he continued to ask me how my day had been and what my weekend plans were. After just a few seconds of chatting with Jose, I started to feel my own energy and grocery shopping mood, which is usually pretty low, begin to lift. Jose had given me a shot of vitamin energy.

Jose looked to be around the age of 65 and had what I'd term a zest for life. When I asked him his age, he replied, "Eighty-five years young!" I couldn't believe it! "So, what's your secret?" I asked. His smile grew a little wider and he said, "Sonny, never let anyone tell you to slow down. Do what you want to do. Also, no matter what, know that things always work out in the end." What powerful advice. After he handed over my grocery bags, I told him how much I appreciated our chat. As I headed to the door, he called to me, lifting his hand and pointing one finger to his head saying, "It's all about this. It's about your attitude in life!"

Walking to my car, I felt like I had just spoken to maybe the most enlightened person I'd ever met – a bag packer at my local supermarket. You see, that is exactly my point. You just never know where inspiration is going to come from. Also, as I like to point out, when we open conversations with total strangers, regardless of what they do for a living or where we are, we can learn so much about life.

My friend, never underestimate the power of a small compliment, smile or simple word of advice. Since that day, I look forward to visiting my local supermarket because I get to see Jose. His example of a winning attitude and mindset is one for us all to take notice of. To some, the task of packing bags might seem like a boring and insignificant job, but Jose proved that regardless of what you do, you have the power to change people's lives. I can promise you that Jose's sole purpose isn't packing groceries; rather it is having a positive impact on the lives of people lucky enough to be around him. He is certainly doing that at the supermarket.

---

*Like Jose, regardless of our ages or
current status, we all have the power
to make a difference in other people's lives!
Find the little – and big – daily ways
you can elevate others.
Bonus: It will elevate you, too.*

Chapter 34

Positive Attitude
Has No Age Limits

One of the most inspirational people I have ever met is the great Nick Bollettieri. When I think of Nick, I instantly think of one word: energy. Nick, an American, is probably the most famous tennis coach ever. He pioneered the concept of the tennis boarding school, his IMG Academy, in Bradenton, Florida. He has trained and coached some of the world's best tennis players, including 10 world #1s. In 2014 he was inducted to the International Tennis Hall of Fame and in the following year, he became the first white man to be inducted into the Black Tennis Hall of Fame. Born in Pelham, New York, to immigrant Italian parents, Nick served with the United States Army, attaining the rank of first lieutenant. He then progressed into coaching. I've had the privilege and honor to get to know Nick over the years, and when I see him, it never ceases to amaze me how much energy and zest for life he has.

Nick gets up each morning at 4:00 a.m. and is the first to arrive on campus, usually before 5:00. He starts each day in the gym and after a quick breakfast goes out to the court. After lunch, it's back to the court to teach until 5:30 p.m. Then he and his wife Cindi pick up their sons from baseball practice. After dinner he works on emails, returns calls and prepares for the next day. Bedtime is around 11 p.m. On Saturdays he works at the academy in the morning before playing 36 holes of golf. Sunday is reserved for his family. Nick also travels a ridiculous number of miles per year. The man's energy is limitless, and, oh, did I mention he is 88 years of age this year?

When I bumped into Nick recently at the Miami Open, I asked him what his secret is. Nick leaned in and said, "Allistair, it's all about your attitude. Your attitude is everything in life." Nick is indeed an example of self-discipline and a never-say-quit attitude. What an amazing example for all of us.

I know many people who are only in their 30s and 40s who have already stopped living. They are stuck in the rearview mirror, looking back at the good old days. Many of these folks look exhausted, uninspired and defeated. They complain that they feel old and they moan that their body aches all the time. These individuals have convinced themselves that their best days are already behind them. They become the words they keep telling themselves when they could instead use that energy looking forward to what could still come. Look around. People who say they feel younger than their calendar years seem to live longer. Self-talk is powerful – choose yours well.

Another great example of a winning attitude is author Babette Hughes. Babette wrote her first book, *Searching for Vivian,* in her 80s. Babette, who is now 94, has written three more books and is a *Huffington Post* contributor. When asked about her age and how she was able to stay relevant, Vivian answered, "We are brainwashed by society and certain beliefs. I don't conform to those. It doesn't matter what age you are because it all comes down to your attitude. Anyone of any age can still make a significant difference to the world."

Just like Nick and Babette, we all have a choice. We can be limited by our excuses about our age, we can be influenced by what society thinks or believes, or we can choose to have a winning attitude and mindset toward life. Take charge of your mind and you'll discover that anything is possible.

———————————————————

You're never too old to set a new goal or dream a new dream.

– C. S. Lewis

Chapter 35

With a Winner's Attitude Anything Is Possible

L ife is all about choices. With this in mind, I believe that there are two kinds of people in the world. There are those who have chosen to see their challenging backgrounds as a lesson in life that gives them the resilience and grit to eventually succeed. Then there are those with the same circumstances who use them as an excuse why they didn't succeed. Former first lady Michelle Obama once said, "You should never view your challenges as a disadvantage. Instead, it's important that your experience facing and overcoming adversity is actually one of your biggest advantages."

Some can stay in the same state of mind (blaming their past), while others choose to live in gratitude and make the most of today. Jim Carrey, star in *The Mask* and *Ace Ventura,* used to be homeless. When he was 15, he had to drop out of school to support his family. His father was an unemployed musician and as the family went from lower middle class to poor, they all ended up living in a van. Carrey didn't let this stop him from achieving his dream of becoming a comedian. With a determined mindset and winner's attitude, Carrey went from having his dad drive him to comedy clubs in Toronto to starring in mega-blockbusters and being known as one of the best comedic actors of an era.

Professional surfer Bethany Hamilton started surfing when she was just a child. At age 13, an almost deadly shark attack resulted in the loss of her left arm. With a passion to succeed and a winner's attitude, she was back on her surfboard one month later. Two years later she won first place in the Explorer Women's Division of the National Scholastic Surfing Association National Championships. Bethany has gone on to have an incredibly successful career. What grit and resilience!

British entrepreneur and billionaire, Richard Branson has dyslexia. In fact, he was a pretty bad student. Instead of giving up or having a defeatist attitude, Branson used the power of his personality to drive him to success. Today Branson, known for developing Virgin Records and many of its more technologically advanced spinoffs, is currently the fourth richest man in the United Kingdom. Talk about persistence!

Multiple Olympic gold medalist gymnast Simone Biles didn't have the easiest upbringing. She was born to a mother who struggled with substance abuse, and was adopted and raised by her grandparents. Simone's journey in gymnastics began by accident. Her outdoor school field trip was canceled, so the teacher chose an indoor one instead – a gymnastics studio. Upon seeing her moves, someone from the gym wrote a note home asking if her parents would consider letting her join the gym. Fast forward, Simone, who stands at 4'9", is today the most decorated gymnast ever. Now that's taking a lemon of a beginning and making lemonade!

Though he is one of the world's richest men and founder of Microsoft, Bill Gates' first business failed. Yes, the richest person in the whole world couldn't make any money on his first company. Traf-O-Data, with the goal of reading traffic tapes and processing the data, failed miserably. But it didn't stop Gates from becoming successful. He was determined.

Kayla Harrison endured a rough upcoming in her sport of judo. At age 13, she became depressed and suicidal when she was sexually assaulted by her judo coach. However, she overcame this, going on to be the first American to win gold medals in judo at the 2012 and 2016 Olympic Games. Today, she continues her career, winning more gold medals and becoming an inspirational speaker as well as an advocate and speaker against child sexual abuse.

Albert Einstein didn't speak until he was four years old, but he was actually a genius. Founding father Benjamin Franklin dropped out of school at age ten. Walt Disney was fired from his job for not being creative enough! (I bet that boss spent time kicking himself around when Disney created Mickey Mouse not too many years later.) J.K. Rowling was rejected by publishers 27 times before being signed. The list can go on and on of people who either came from a disadvantaged background or had one or a multitude of failures and disappointments.

When something bad happens to you, you have two choices. You can either let it destroy you or you can let it strengthen you. All the people above chose their attitude and decided to turn their disadvantaged pasts, challenges or tragedies into successful outcomes and futures. The common denominator among them was a steely determination to find a greater purpose in life and to succeed. Sooner or later they chose to focus all their energy on achieving their dreams and goals. They adopted a winner's attitude and mindset, and they used their past as a deeper motivation to succeed instead of an excuse not to.

*Remembering these role models,
use your past disadvantages
as daily motivation to succeed.*

SECTION 6

EMPATHY

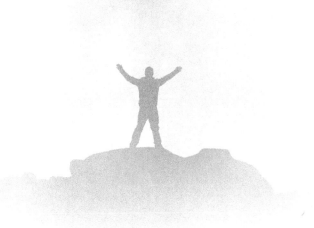

Chapter 36

EQ Can Take You Further than IQ

IQ, Intelligence Quotient, is the number that indicates a person's intelligence level. Fact is, you can't improve your IQ. But the good news is that you can improve something that's way more beneficial – your EQ. EQ, or emotional intelligence, refers to the ability to identify and manage one's own emotions, as well as to identify and work with the emotions of others. In practical terms, it means being aware that emotions can drive our behavior and impact people (positively and negatively) and learning how to manage those emotions, especially when we are under pressure. That's why it's fair to say that people who exude a winner's attitude and mindset have better control of their own emotions and a clearer understanding of others' emotions.

I first heard about emotional intelligence several years ago at in a bookstore in the Atlanta airport. I picked up *Emotional intelligence 2.0* by Dr. Travis Bradberry and finished it by the time I got to Toronto. It has been a game changer! I was so inspired that from the moment I stepped off the aircraft I was already putting what I had read into practice.

Emotional intelligence is one of the most important elements to having a winning attitude and mindset. A study from the Carnegie Institute of Technology found that 85% of a company's financial success is predicated on human skills, while statistics from Harvard and Stanford show an interestingly similar finding that 85-87% of an individual's success comes from their personal skills. The reality is that clients and customers would rather do business with people they like and trust even when someone else might be offering a better product at a lower price.

In the years since that flight to Toronto, I have continued to work on my EQ. If I'm being honest with myself, I wasn't always the most sociable person and would at times struggle in group projects or environments. Only later did I realize that the majority of people want to work with people they really like and connect with. At the end of the day, success is about the relationships you build and nurture. I wish I'd realized earlier in my life and career just how important emotional intelligence really is. In fact, the more I think about it, the more it comes down to two simple words: kindness and empathy. I believe that those who really get ahead today are those with great emotional intelligence and who are just nice people. Anyway, who wants to work with or be associated with a jerk?

You probably know people who are masters at managing their emotions, and I'm sure you know those who fail miserably at it, too. I see both every day. No, I'm not judging; I'm simply stating what I witness and experience on a daily basis. Those who are able to manage their emotions don't get uptight and panic or get angry in stressful situations. They don't let the raging chimp (with thanks to British psychologist Steve Peters for his book *The Chimp Paradox*) get out of control. Instead, they have the ability to look at a problem and calmly find a solution. They are excellent decision makers and are willing to look at themselves honestly. They know how to take criticism well, and they know how to use it to improve their own performance. Aren't these the people you prefer to spend time around? Don't you want to be this kind of person?

Ever wonder why some people seem to get those lucky breaks and get ahead in life more often than others who have more skills, knowledge or experience? It's got a lot to do with simply knowing how to get along with others better. They handle stress well and don't expect others to handle it better than they do. You obviously don't need a Harvard or Yale education to learn this.

If you've got the education and experience to get ahead, but it's not happening, maybe what you need to do is work on your personality more than on your career-related knowledge. Hey, I did. It is one of the best decisions I ever made, and I'm happy to say that it's working! The good news is that while some people have a natural penchant for it, others can learn it by example. Today, when I see a great leader, teacher, manager or coach, the first thing I see is someone with great emotional intelligence.

Ok, so great, Allistair, how do I gain more emotional intelligence? Well, for one thing, be more mindful of others. Pause before you speak; don't blurt out everything you're thinking. If it could in any way be hurtful or unhelpful, then maybe it's not the ideal thing to say. Be aware of the timing of saying things. Also, don't expect better behavior from others than you do from yourself.

Consider learning more about these concepts. There are many great resources both on the internet and in book stores. This can be a game changer for you, too! People with a winning attitude and mindset get this.

Signs that you have high emotional intelligence – you

- Smile more
- Forgive more
- Have patience
- Listen to understand, not to reply
- Remember people's names
- Don't interrupt others

- Don't respond to negativity
- Are able to control your anger
- Are grateful and have empathy
- Are respectful and have manners
- Respect differences and other opinions
- Don't gossip about others
- Gather all the facts first
- Don't judge quickly
- Show appreciation
- Are open-minded
- Prefer to be silent than to engage in drama
- Are interested in others more than yourself

People who consistently exude a winner's attitude and mindset have better control over their emotions and a clearer understanding of others, and they enjoy greater financial and personal benefits. You have nothing to lose from trying it!

Chapter 37

Relationships Create Opportunity

You want the good life. The visions are dancing in your head. And there are other visions. You imagine the jobs you will apply and be selected for, the resumes and the interviews you will deal with, the practice sessions you will grind through, the work you will do on your way to the top. Back up for a moment. The road to success is not just about vehicles, but also about people you meet along the way. Some of these people – sometimes the least likely ones – will open doors for you. More importantly, they will enrich the quality of your life immeasurably.

Unfortunately, one area where a lot of people, especially those less experienced, make mistakes is in the job hunt. They ask about what they are going to get – benefits, vacation days and first raise. This is a huge mistake. Those who get ahead focus on investing in long-term relationships first.

Another common mistake is misplaced concentration on the pursuit of growth and success in careers instead of building what really matters most – again, longer and stronger relationships. People want to skip the process and get quickly to where the supposed rewards are. Don't let this happen to you. Relationships bring enjoyment both day to day and long term. In addition, the people you associate with now can connect you to positions and successes (you guessed it) both day to day and long term. Win-win.

Now make no mistake, it's not as simple as the old saying, "It's not what you know; it's who you know." In order for people to be willing to recommend you, you first have to have the knowledge and the skills required. Competent people are not going to jeopardize their own reputations by vouching for incompetence. So assuming you do have the requisite knowledge and experience, the question is, how are you going to get ahead of others who also do? The answer is Relationships. When you focus on building and nurturing relationships instead of only trying to build an impressive resume, you give yourself the greatest chance to grow your network and create even more opportunities.

But relationships are worth much more than opening doors to professional success. In an 80-year Harvard study, researchers concluded that it wasn't money, fame, material possessions or achievements that made people happy; it was, in fact, close relationships.

Let people know that you are sincerely interested in them as individuals. Over time this becomes the foundation to all trust. You can't fake it. To emphasize an important point I mentioned earlier, in the long run, even if what you said is forgotten, how you made others feel is remembered. This is something the best influencers in their fields know well.

I wish I had known it in my younger years. About 15 years ago I transitioned my focus from being work driven to being people driven. The result? A way happier me, not to mention a way busier and more productive me. Today, I have an abundance of exciting projects and work that have provided me with fulfilling opportunities. And from these opportunities has serendipitously come more financial freedom.

You can't succeed if you don't have the right people around you. It takes teamwork. Maybe you are one of those people who feel that you're not great at meeting new people, that you are introverted or shy. Well, I'm going to be brutally honest with you now; if you keep telling yourself that, you'll be holding yourself back from realizing your unlimited potential and personal greatness. You are missing out on an abundance of things life has to offer. Even if you have the goal of meeting or making conversation with just one new person a day, that will increase your network by 365 people. That gives you 365 better chances of getting to where you want to be. But you have to take the first step. For example, when you check out at the grocery store, say thank you to the cashier and the bagger, and use their names. Expand from there.

Most successful people I speak with tell me that one of the main factors in their becoming leaders in their fields is the relationships they've built over the years. The more hands you shake, the more relationships and opportunities you make.

Meeting someone and soon thereafter asking for a job or an opportunity is not the best approach. Relationships are about trust, and trust takes time. The key is to form relationships before you need them. Let like-ability be your best ability.

Consistently think long term. The relationships you build with people who are strangers now become the foundation of your success and growth in your future.

The more hands you shake,
the more opportunities and
relationships you make.

Chapter 38

Let People Know They Matter

B ill Bullard, former Michigan state senator, once said, "The highest form of knowledge is empathy." And I believe that it is one of the most meaningful and powerful traits a person can have. Empathetic people are kind and thoughtful. They put themselves into the shoes of other people – to feel, understand and see things from their point of view. Because empathetic people try to experience the emotions, thoughts and feelings of others, they treat others as they want to be treated. What does empathy look like?

After a delayed flight coming from Los Angeles, I landed at JFK in New York. It was 12:00 p.m. on a Saturday afternoon and I was scheduled to speak at the Grand Hyatt at 3:00 p.m. Yep, I know, pushing it real fine. I was pretty tired from the trip and the three-hour time difference coming from the west coast, but I had to put that aside as I was about to speak to well over 300 people. On arriving at the hotel, I saw that the check-in line had around 30 people and the lobby was packed with others waiting for their rooms to come available. After traveling for nine hours (door to door), all I wanted to do was get a shower and a quick lie down before I was due to speak.

After about 25 minutes in line, I found myself facing five receptionists who all looked under pressure and overwhelmed. I approached the next available one, Sophie, who took a deep breath and said, "Good afternoon, sir, and welcome to the Grand Hyatt." I could see and feel that Sophie was exhausted. I greeted her with, "Wow, it's extra busy today, isn't it? I just want to say how much we appreciate you and the team right now. You're doing a fantastic job!" Sophie looked up from her computer screen and smiled. She probably hadn't heard that all day. Sophie asked me how my day was going, and I told her about my trip and the fact I had to speak in less than two hours. She explained that the wait was about an hour and a half. I said, "No problem, I completely understand, and I appreciate everything you are doing. But if there's a small chance of getting a room quicker, I'd be the happiest guy on earth." She smiled again and said she'd do the best she could. I smiled back and thanked her once again.

I sat down with the irritated throng, but made sure I stayed in sight of Sophie. It was probably only 10 minutes before I felt a tap on the shoulder. Sophie had my room key in her hand and wished me a pleasant stay. I asked her how she was able to perform this miracle so fast. She replied, "You are the first guest who has asked me how I was today and told me that I'm appreciated, so thank you." This was empathy and emotional intelligence working at its finest. Happy to say I got a much needed shower and a 20-minute nap before my presentation that afternoon.

Empathy is the ability to communicate and be a better leader by understanding others' thoughts, views, and feelings. When we improve our empathy, we also become better humans.

Here is something I've learned in the people business: People need to know they matter. They need to know what they do is noticed and that their efforts are appreciated. In fact, people need to know they matter regardless of what they do or who they are. This is one of the key reasons that empathic people succeed more than others. It's not that they know more, but rather that they feel things more. They are more dialed into people than into projects.

Highly empathetic people sense the emotions of those around them, and have the ability to tap into those same emotions within themselves. In essence, they "become" the person they're empathizing with by truly *experiencing* other people's emotions.

So how can we become better at empathy? Well, Professor Simon Baron Cohen puts it quite simply: "Empathy is a skill like any other human skill. If you practice it often enough, you can get better at it."

Here are 4 tips to become a more empathetic person:

1. Listen More than You Speak

Great communicators are 80% listeners and 20% talkers; however, most of us speak at least twice as much as we listen. It's easy to get so caught up explaining something that we fail to stop and consider what the other person might be thinking or feeling. Try to commit your undivided attention to the conversation and listen so you can really understand. When we listen, we learn. The best leaders, managers, coaches, etc. are great listeners.

2. Don't Make Negative Assumptions

Here's why assumptions are dangerous to empathy: When we make a negative assumption, we rarely do a good job relating to the problem the other person is facing. As a result, the connection we try to make is likely inaccurate. To have negative assumptions is to harbor preconceived notions that are not based on true knowledge or experience. Often we use these assumptions as shortcuts to solve a problem. But when we do that, we don't see the full picture.

3. Challenge yourself

Undertake challenging experiences which push you outside your comfort zone. For example, learn a new skill, such as a musical instrument, hobby, or foreign language. Develop a new professional competency. Why? Aside from helping your brain, doing things like these will humble you, and humility is a key enabler of empathy.

4. Get feedback

Ask for feedback about your relationship skills (listening) from family, friends, and colleagues – and then check in with them periodically to see how you're doing. Feedback is what makes us better. When we take feedback well and put it into practice, we are able to grow.

Remember: Empathy is a *skill*, which means it can be *learned*. At first, this whole practice may feel unnatural and a little awkward. Don't worry: Like any skill, empathy feels a little cumbersome at first. But the more you do it, the more natural it will become and the less conscious thought it will demand. Keep at it and I promise you'll get there; and the relationships you'll build and connections you'll form will be worth it. Empathy leads to stronger, more meaningful relationships. It leads to success in the workplace. Last but not least, empathy leads to your own better health and quality of life.

---

*Empathy is the ability
to consistently communicate and lead well
by understanding others' thoughts,
views and feelings.*

Chapter 39

Know Thyself

Developing a winning attitude and mindset involves developing emotional intelligence. One of the best books I've read on the subject is Daniel Goleman's *Emotional Intelligence.* In his book Goleman discusses the importance of two particular abilities necessary to succeed in life. The first is knowing yourself, and the second is having empathy, a better understanding of others.

I'm sure it will come as little surprise when I tell you that people who know themselves well and are able to understand the feelings of others are more likeable and better able to connect with others. These people usually have higher levels of emotional intelligence than others. Those who have a lower level of emotional intelligence find it difficult to process their own feelings and are unskilled in engaging with the feelings of others.

It is important to know that IQ (intelligence quotient) and emotional intelligence are not related. There are unfortunately people who are academically gifted but have no idea about empathizing with their fellow human beings. They may have no idea why they are being passed over for opportunities that less gifted people are getting.

We are emotional creatures who sometimes let our emotions run wild. Keeping a winning attitude and mindset includes the ability to better control our own emotions and being able to not say the thing that could ruin a relationship or cause a problem. Emotional self-awareness is the foundation on which emotional intelligence is built. I must admit, in my own journey to improving myself and developing a winning attitude, I have felt the incredible power and benefit of having more self-awareness. It has opened my eyes and helped me grow as a human being.

As I noted earlier, even though my job involves public speaking and consulting, I didn't always have the best social skills. I wouldn't have called myself a complete introvert growing up, but I did like to be by myself a lot. In fact, over the years working in the human performance field, I've realized that you can tell a lot about someone's personality by the kind of activities or sports they do. Mine were running and biking, which involved many long, lonely hours on the road. Later in life, I discovered that one of the keys to success was the ability to socialize and build relationships – at that time, not a natural thing for me to do. I had to work on it, and it's still a work in progress. I discovered that most things in life are connected to relationships.

When others see that we are empathetic, they know that we are caring and connected. Marshall B. Rosenberg, psychologist and author of *Nonviolent Communication,* writes that people who develop their capacity for empathy become more compassionate toward themselves and others. It is a win-win attitude because empathic people then attract other caring and compassionate people to themselves.

Knowing yourself and spending time in becoming a better you is probably one of the most worthwhile things a person can do. It's a never ending journey and process. I encourage you to spend time in self-reflection, developing empathy and compassion. When you do, you will discover that having the power of understanding your own feelings and those of others is indeed incredible power.

Seek first to understand,
then to be understood.

– Dr. Stephen Covey

Chapter 40

People with Winning Attitudes Are Givers

A valuable truth I learned at an early age was that it's good to help other people. It feels awesome. My mother taught my three older brothers and me that it's better to give than to receive. My amazing mother was (and still is) all about giving back to the community by helping at church soup kitchens and local charities. One of her unforgettable examples of kindness occurred when I was around 11 years old. I was playing in the garden while my mother was tending the plants. A poor and frail man came to the gate and asked for water. My mother not only got him water, but food, too. She told me, *"Never deny anyone food or a drink ever."* It has stuck with me to this very day. Every time I go out of town, I pack a few shirts or wristbands to give out as gifts. I deeply feel that giving, no matter how small, is closely linked to gratitude and a winning attitude.

Opportunities to give are everywhere. One that might appeal to you is giving your time or sharing your knowledge or expertise with younger or lesser experienced people in your industry or community. I love to share like this and see how I've helped others grow. I have been blessed to have such a wonderful career, experienced so much with so many incredible people a lot smarter than I am, and so it's natural that I feel obliged to give back. When it comes to a career path, I believe that

- You first you get paid for what you do
- Then you get paid for what you know
- Then you get paid for who you grow

We evolve. Our purpose changes.

The first part of my career, in my 20s, I started in the fitness and sports performance industry. Then in my 30s I knew a bit more and got to move up the ladder in terms of better jobs, projects and offers. Now in my 40s, I am fortunate enough to get paid for sharing what I know through consulting, writing and speaking. When I get to share my knowledge and witness others grow, I feel a great sense of achievement and inner joy. I want to make a difference.

The greatest turning point for me came from changing my mindset from a taking one to a giving one. Early on, when I met someone, I thought about what I could get from them. Later, when I adopted a more "what can I do for this person?" approach and mentality, things changed dramatically: internally and externally, and in relationships, finances and opportunities. I learned to become a better listener. When I meet someone now, I listen carefully to see how I can help them.

People with winning attitudes love to give and help in whatever way possible. We all have something we can share with the world. You don't need to be famous or rich to inspire others. You just have to show you care. Even just a word of wisdom or the smallest of compliments can help change someone's path, and even life, forever.

Making it a habit to find ways to help others improves your own life in addition to theirs. Be a giver.

SECTION 7

PERSPECTIVE

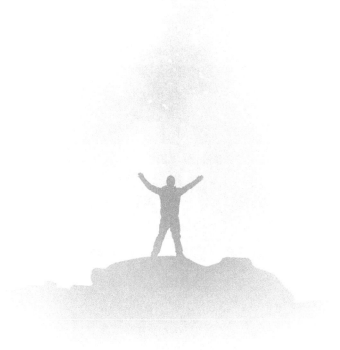

Chapter 41

Winners Give
It GAS Each Day

One practice that has had a profound influence on my life is a daily habit I call GAS – gratitude, appreciation and self-reflection. Incorporating this powerful three-part routine into my life has helped me be happier and more fulfilled. And it can do the same for you.

The first thing on waking each morning I focus on gratitude. I immediately think of two or three things I'm grateful for. At first I had a sticky note next to my bed saying "gratitude." This helped me create the habit. There are many things in life to be grateful for that we take for granted; for example, our health, our family and friends, our warm bed, the sun shining through the window, our car, or the opportunity to get out there and chase our goals for another day. Already before I put a foot on the floor, I feel a positive energy and enthusiasm to get after my day and chase my greater purpose.

Along the same lines, some people like to write a gratitude list; it is another great way to keep in mind the good things in our lives, which can become so easy to take for granted. In a study from Southern Methodist University in Dallas, Texas, an institution that I've consulted to in the past, a group examined the extraordinarily positive impact of gratitude on people's overall well-being. A few hundred people were split into three groups, all of whom agreed to write in a diary at the end of each day for the duration of the study. The first group received no instructions as to what to record, so they could write about whatever happened during the day, either positive or negative. The second group was instructed to write only about unpleasant experiences they'd had throughout the day. The third group was instructed to write only about things that they were grateful for.

The results of the study showed that the third group, those who wrote their daily gratitudes at the end of each day, experienced higher overall levels of alertness, enthusiasm, determination, optimism and energy. But wait, there's more! The third group also experienced less depression and stress and was more likely to help others and make greater progress toward their personal goals. What a broad spectrum of priceless results! And here's another big one: People in the third group – just through the luck of getting assigned to that group – *developed* a more positive attitude. That means that you don't have to be a naturally optimistic person; you can choose to become one – choose to find the positives each day – and reap huge life-long benefits. The desire to have more in your career, relationships, bank account, etc. can be quite motivating, but thinking about what you already have, and expressing gratitude for it, can enhance your life in ways you can't imagine.

The second act I perform on a daily basis is to show appreciation to people who add to my life. What does this mean? It means that I express gratitude to my neighbor who is always friendly and helpful, to doormen who are ready to lend a hand, to my colleagues, to the person packing my grocery bags at the store and to the maintenance man who keeps the restroom nice and clean; if we pay attention, the list is long. Doing this reminds me how fortunate I am. We all know that showing appreciation to others, whether by words or actions, is an act of love and kindness because everyone wants to feel special and appreciated. If I get to cheer up someone else's day, even just for a small moment, it's well worth the effort. In fact, I get a kick out of seeing people smile when I tell them that I truly appreciate them. I feel the energy shift up another level.

The third part of my routine is to finish my day in self-reflection. Self-reflection is the process of looking inside yourself and bringing your attention to what's happening in your life in a mindful and open-minded way. It's about creating self-awareness. I ask myself these three simple questions:

1. What did I do well today?
2. What could I have done better today?
3. Who did I make better today?

Asking myself these questions each evening before turning off the light has helped me look inward and see if I am making progress to fulfilling my greater purpose and vision for my life. Self-reflection is one of the best ways to become more emotionally intelligent. It's not always easy, as at times you will have to face up to some things that you either regret saying or are ashamed of doing, but it's when we address things instead of pushing them away that we become better human beings.

As I write this, I am spending a few days at a Buddhist temple in Brisbane, Australia. One of my best friends, Brad, recommended it – thanks, mate! This is something I would not have done in the past. I used to be closed minded. Thankfully, over time I've become more open-minded and am able to benefit from additional ideas and experiences in life. I am not religious, but I do believe in God, and also in some of the principles of recognized religions. For example, Buddhism teaches gratitude, love and kindness. The head monk at this temple, Hui, is a font of knowledge, and I make the most of every chance I get to learn from him. I told him about my GAS theory, and he gave it his seal of approval.

GAS up each day. Start by practicing gratitude in the morning before you hop out of bed. Then aim to show appreciation throughout the day. Finally, end each day by self-reflecting on the day you've had. This is a great way to develop a winner's attitude and mindset.

———————————

No one who achieves success
does it without the help of others.
The wise and confident
acknowledge this help with gratitude.

– Alfred N. Whitehead

Chapter 42

Winners Have a Vision

Winners know where they are going. They have a vision and they see that vision every day. They have direction and a destination.

As you might recall, I had Bob Bowman on my podcast. Bob is the long-time coach of the most decorated Olympian of all time, swimmer Michael Phelps. This is what Bob had to say about having a vision:

> You need a vision of where you want to go, what you want to do and who you want to be someday down the road. Think creatively about what it is you want out of life and where it is you want to go. Dream, fantasize and allow yourself to suspend your beliefs to envision the life you want. Put your visions in writing. Remember that the vision should excite you and make you jump out of bed every morning. You need to live your vision daily. You have to incorporate the above qualities every day of your life and keep your mission at the top of your daily agenda.

Bob absolutely nails it. Success becomes routine when you have a routine. Map out the day and try to stick to a daily schedule that pushes you forward. Go about the task at hand professionally, and set high standards for yourself. The more consistent you are with your daily work, the more likely you will succeed. Keep taking the steps on a daily basis, ratchet up the pressure and challenge yourself to do a little more each day.

When I ask people what their greater vision or purpose is, you'd be surprised that the majority can't tell me exactly what it is. I always tell them that it's hard for me to help them if they don't know exactly what it is or where they are heading. It's a bit like driving your car without a destination. You need clarity on where you are headed before you get started. Along the way, it's important to have intermediate goals that let you know that you are on track. If you don't develop your own vision, you allow other people and circumstances to direct the course of your life; greatness is about being in control of your own destiny. When you truly believe in what you are doing, it shows and it pays. Winners in life are those who are excited about their greater purpose and where they are going.

6 Questions to Help You Discover Your Vision

1. What is close to your heart and really matters to you in life?
2. What would bring you more joy in your life?
3. What do you really care about?
4. What are your talents? What's special about you?
5. What would you like to have more of in your life?
6. What legacy would you like to leave behind?

To create your vision, begin by identifying your core values, your passions, what you believe to be your purpose, and how you envision your life. Set the intermediate goals to touch on along the way, the check points that help you stay on track. Having a vision and setting goals are essential to your success, not optional. No greatness can be achieved without taking these steps.

One final note here is that you shouldn't expect a clear and well-defined vision overnight – envisioning your life and determining the course you will follow requires reflection. Take time to think about what it is you really want.

5 Benefits of Having a Vision for Your Life

1. It gives meaning and purpose to what you're doing
2. It provides clarity
3. It provides focus
4. It motivates you through challenging times
5. It provides validation and the feeling of profound accomplishment when you succeed

Your vision should excite and ignite you, especially through times of adversity. It will keep you moving forward if you focus on it every day.

All great things first started
with having a vision and a greater purpose.

Chapter 43

Put on Your Own Face Mask First

Success by itself won't bring you happiness, especially if you have illness that you allowed to happen. Ask anyone who has lost their health, and they will tell you that they would pay any amount of money to have it back again. Good health is a sacred possession. As selfish as it may sound, taking care of your health needs to be at the top of your priority list. If you don't take care of that, how can you expect to take care of others? Last year I took over 100 flights, and on every one, the flight attendant advised, "Put on your own face mask before helping someone else." I believe that it's great passenger advice – and a metaphor for life.

When asked about the most important traits to being happy and successful, British billionaire, entrepreneur and founder of Virgin Airlines, Sir Richard Branson said, "Having good health is the key to happiness, and happiness is the key to success." Wise words from someone who has been at the top of his game for well over three decades. Branson went on to say, "I'm wealthy, successful and connected because I am happy. And I am happy because I make my health, fitness and mindfulness a priority, each and every day."

It's evident that Sir Richard exudes a winning attitude and mindset when it comes to health, happiness and success. What he understands is that you can't function to your capacity if you don't tend to your health with positive energy. When asked his top tip for productivity, he replied, "You need to exercise and work out. It's that simple." The founder of the many Virgin Group companies takes time to get active no matter how busy he is, and believes that rather than being a dent in his schedule, exercise enables him to power through an extra four hours of work a day. The most important aspect of his workout routine, Branson emphasizes, is consistency.

Taking care of your health is key in living a wonderful life. The connection between the mind and body is huge. Having a positive attitude in life includes the conscious decision to be proactive about your health. Studies have shown that healthy outlooks also reduce risks to our well-being, especially after adversity or negative life events. Those who say they don't have time for exercise or working out are basically saying they don't value themselves or those they care for enough to work at staying healthy. Even just 20 minutes a day can make all the difference! Remember, you are not really going to be much good for anyone else in your life if you are depleted, lacking energy, or in a state of constant irritability. There is a great quote that says, "Those who don't find time for exercise now will have to find time for illness later." It's true; when you don't get the balance right in life – working long hours without down time for self-care – you will pay for it later.

I start my day by choosing my health first. I get my exercise done first thing in the morning, even when I'm on the road. I usually get up around 5:30 a.m. and hit the hotel gym, go for a run, or work out in the room; I find a way to get it done. Leaving it for later in the day can be tricky as I don't always know how the day will pan out. By tackling my mental and physical health when I get up, I feel I am priming my mind and body for success right out of the gate.

I am frequently asked, "What are the best exercises or equipment to get the best results?" My advice? Do what you enjoy the most – be it yoga, CrossFit, rollerblading, swimming, biking, tennis, etc. The reason is simple – when you do what you enjoy most, you will want to do more of it. For example, if I were to tell you to run, but you absolutely detest running, I can promise that your exercise regimen wouldn't last long. Do what you love to do and you will keep your motivation longer. I used to be a critic of CrossFit, but over the years, I've seen what a positive impact and transformation it's had on people's lives – both in social interaction and in self-confidence.

My best advice when it comes to getting in shape is not to focus on what exercises to do (because there are no magic exercises), but rather to focus on the environment you love to be in. Find your tribe, people you love to be around, and go work out! The results will come when you take your mind away from what your body is doing and put it into the enjoyment of being around a group of people with a shared interest who are spurring each other on. The goal here is to get in at least 20 minutes a day of movement. Whatever it is, just get out there and commit to it!

Make your health priority number one. If you want to realize your purpose and live a productive, happy and prosperous life, you first need to invest in your health. Saying you don't have the time is saying, "it doesn't' matter enough to me." You will find time for the things that are important to you.

No matter what age you are or what shape you're in, fact is, there is no better time to start than now. It doesn't get any easier the longer you let it go, believe me. The secret is to get going and to build the habit. Without health, it's hard to accomplish what you want in life.

Consistent attention to your health is truly key to your happiness and success.

Chapter 44

Winners Embrace the Journey

ere's the good news about failure – it's temporary. Here's the bad news about success – it, too, is temporary. So, don't allow yourself to take the highs and lows of outcomes too seriously. Those who do eventually pay the price. Achievements are great confirmation of the work you've put in, but each one moves to the rearview mirror, and the journey continues. Embrace your journey. It's not just the achievements you earn but the effort you give day in and day out along the way that will make you who you become and determine the quality of your continuing journey and your future.

I have witnessed it all too often, in sports and in other careers, that people get so wrapped up in the outcome that they forget to enjoy the process. They live and die for success and failure when, if they instead focused on the process, they would find real joy in the journey. Gaining confidence is about putting the outcome aside. Everything you do in life – good, bad or indifferent – is a lesson that can give you confidence. Those with a winner's attitude and mindset focus on what they can control, and what is within their control is the process, not the outcome.

Progress is never a straight line up. The truth about progress is that it's messy. It is where the resistance occurs and fights against you for a period of time. Making progress is about working through the mess and learning to embrace it along the way. The mess is where you experience the struggle, doubt, confusion, frustration and a feeling of "I'm not getting anywhere." It is by enduring and working through this difficult space that we eventually experience the growth. This is when we see the line of progress become more steadily upward. Winners get this.

Of course developing or having a winner's attitude and mindset doesn't mean that you don't at times question yourself. That's normal. In fact, I've had the privilege of working with some of the world's highest performers and most positive people, and I can tell you that they do indeed experience doubts along their personal journey to greatness. Some of them have embraced it better than others, but the great ones who have understood the process have gotten there much sooner than those who fought it. You see, the secret is to learn to understand the process of the journey, to navigate the bumps that are an inevitable part of the process and finally to appreciate and embrace the process.

Achieving anything of significance requires an all-in commitment, relentless effort and countless hours of hard work. There will be mistakes and failures. There will be disappointments and challenges. There will be setbacks and fear. But these are what embracing the journey is all about. Those with a winner's attitude and mindset see adversity and setbacks as great opportunities to grow and learn. When you take advantage of these challenges, you develop grit and resilience – two qualities that every champion possesses. In life, things happen to you for reasons, good and bad. Sometimes we get to understand them only much later on.

Achieving your own personal greatness is about having the courage to set big goals and then go after them with all you've got. But great things take time. It's important to practice patience along the way but still be consistent and persistent in your everyday actions. Don't beat yourself up if you don't have the perfect day, exactly because when you're reaching for greatness, it will be messy and confusing at times. Thomas Edison created 1,000 unsuccessful light bulbs. When asked about his 1,000 failures, he replied that he didn't fail 1,000 times, but that the light bulb was a project with 1,000 steps. Sometimes you just have to go with the flow and trust that tomorrow will be a better day.

Embracing your journey also involves a greater connection with yourself. This is where the benefit of self-awareness comes in. Hard times reveal who you are. Know that when you are struggling, you are progressing. As you gain awareness of yourself, you will enjoy your evolution better and embrace your journey with enthusiasm.

I've discovered that it is those who embrace the messiness who progress faster and go further in life. Those who ignore it, complain about it or try to avoid it never reach their potential. They miss the opportunities to build more grit and resilience. The winners in their fields learn and grow from the good, the bad and the ugly. They see it all as an advantage. They may have struggled with it at first, but they learned that it is important to roll with the punches and believe in the greater long-term vision. That's why it's important to be optimistic. See every mistake, failure, or difficulty as part of life and never allow these problems get the best of you.

Remember, that no one who made it to the top or achieved their personal greatness had a smooth ride. Know that you were made for great things, but you have to keep putting in the daily work, keep hustling, stay positive and stay patient. Appreciate the value of the process.

Last but not least, your journey is unique. Don't compare it with anyone else's. See your challenges as your own personal opportunities. See failures as valuable lessons.

When you consistently embrace the journey with a humble, patient, open and learner's wisdom, you will experience huge growth. This is the approach of a winner's attitude and mindset.

---

*Every journey includes rough spots.
People with a winner's attitude and mindset
focus on the ones they can control
within the process, and embrace the journey
as they learn and grow.*

Chapter 45

Develop an Attitude of Gratitude

People with a winner's attitude start each day in gratitude. Each and every day it's important to be thankful for what we have while we work for what we want. So often I hear people saying things like "when I get that promotion, I'll be happy" or "when I get that car, I'll be happy." Well, they might be happy for a few days or if they're lucky a few weeks, but then it wears off. Happiness is about being present in this moment and being thankful for it. Gratitude is the foundation of happiness. Knowing that there are many who have far less than we have and would trade places with us in an instant, we need to pause and reflect on how fortunate we really are.

True greatness doesn't come to those who fail to appreciate what they have. That's one reason it's important to maintain an attitude of gratitude. Something I believe with all my heart is that there is no real greatness without gratitude.

Author Don Miguel Ruiz said, "The more you practice gratitude, the more you see how much there is to be grateful for." So true. Being grateful is fundamental to living a happy and fulfilled life. It's pretty simple: If you aren't happy with what you have, you aren't happy. The goal is to remain in a constant state of gratitude while continually working toward higher, and higher minded, dreams and goals.

What is gratitude you ask? It's a skill and also an emotion, an action, a mindset and a state of being. Like any other skill, it needs to be practiced. And like any skill, the more you do it, the better you become at it. When you are around grateful people, you feel it instantly, so the more time you spend around other grateful people, the easier it is to maintain and grow this positive frame of mind.

Gratitude is an attitude of being thankful for the life experiences that you have had and the lessons learned from them – good and bad.

It also includes being thankful for friends or family who care about us; never take this for granted. Let me ask you this: When was the last time you told those people within your circle that you love and appreciate them? I mean intentionally, like with a phone call or a text? Today might be a good time.

There is a wonderful law of nature that says three of the things we want most – happiness, freedom and peace of mind – are always attained when we give them away. This is gratitude at its finest – when we show gratitude, we *receive* happiness, freedom and peace of mind.

When we focus on what we are grateful for, we alter not only our perspective but also our state of being. Plato, the Greek philosopher said, "A grateful mind is a great mind, which eventually attracts to itself great things." I believe that it's almost impossible to feel grateful and negative at the same time. When you choose to see the world through a grateful heart, you change how you feel about others in a positive way. Being grateful alters the way we relate to the world and how we see things. It's a choice. Each day and in every moment, we get to choose. Gratitude attracts abundance and it creates healthier and happier relationships. There is unlimited power and potential in gratitude.

I practice gratitude when I wake up each morning. I start by thinking of at least two things I'm grateful for. I try not to repeat them and to challenge myself to think of even the smallest of things I might take for granted; for example, a good night's sleep or the clients or friends I get to see that day.

During the day I aim to live in appreciation, a form of gratitude. I try to stay alert and conscious of all the little things that are happening around me and be thankful. For example, I appreciate the lady serving me at the post office, the waitress at bringing me my coffee at the bakery bar I visit each morning, or a woman in traffic letting me go in front of her. Every day and everywhere we can fill our gratitude tanks. You just have to stay aware of what is going on around you. I used to be so judgmental at times, but I can tell you that introducing this simple exercise into daily practice has dramatically changed everything – especially my energy and general outlook on life.

Another great way of practicing gratitude is journaling. You can do this simple exercise at any time of the day, at the office, at school, or in the evening before bedtime. Simply write down a list of people, things or events you're grateful for that day. The key is to stay consistent and write these down daily. You'll be amazed at the shift that takes place within yourself when you do this exercise, especially when you look back at all the things you've written down over the last few days and weeks. We have much to be grateful for.

Be grateful for what you have
while working for what you want.

Chapter 46

Stay Open-minded

O ne of the keys to achieving a winning attitude and mindset is by staying open-minded. Being open-minded means that, despite your beliefs, you are still willing to hear the views and opinions of others without judging them. From a young age, we are brought up with a certain set of beliefs, values and views instilled in us by our parents. We are also influenced by our environment and the other people around us. However, as we get older we become more curious about the world and how things work. We begin to question things. Maintaining a sense curiosity is priceless.

Keeping an open mind means that we keep learning, evolving and growing. It means being receptive to new ideas as we realize that other people are as much a product of their parents and environments as we are of ours. It is an awareness that we don't have all the answers and so must remain open to learning from others.

One of my social media mentors is someone I've never met, but I still see him as a mentor. He's 82 years of age and his name is George. The reason why he is still so inspiring and relevant today is that he keeps an open mind and keeps learning, evolving and growing – even at his age! He is still interesting to all ages, including teenagers and young athletes from all around the world. He's even on Snapchat! He doesn't let age get in the way of what he's becoming. George has said that you can't stay relevant if you aren't evolving. Instead of being stuck in his old ways, he stays curious. George likes to question things without judgment, but rather with an interest to find out why.

One of the greatest obstacles to becoming someone with a winning attitude and mindset is our ego. It can be hard to reexamine our own ideas, but people with an open mind can do it without feeling threatened. Think for a moment about how much you like or respect the my-way-or-the-highway people you know. Not so much. We don't have to agree with what everyone says, but we can respect their right to their opinions. In fact, I believe that the ability to separate the person from their beliefs, views or opinions is one of the signs of maturity. When you get over that hurdle, then you can learn from almost anybody, regardless of whether you like them or not.

In my third book, *Becoming a Great Team Player,* I touch on the importance of the members of a team staying open-minded and not letting a problematic ego get in the way. In working with many teams – sports, business, academic, etc. – this is one of the main reasons that the best team cultures succeed. Despite diversity in culture, religion, values, sexual preference and backgrounds, members of great teams are able to trust and respect each other and work together effectively. This is possible only through staying open-minded. These teams have a huge edge over teams with self-focused or self-righteous members.

5 Benefits of Staying Open-minded

1. You are more approachable to others

2. You are more empathetic

3. You are viewed as someone worth listening to because your ideas are seen as well thought out

4. Your likeability increases because you are open to listening

5. You open yourself up to learning more

To continually grow,
we must set our ego aside,
stay open-minded and
be willing to learn from others.

SECTION 8

EMBRACE CHANGE

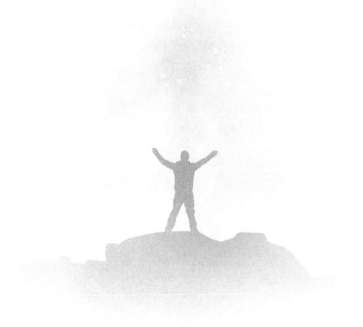

Chapter 47

Redesign Your Life

We get only one life, so why not make it a great one? The person you are today and the place you find yourself are a result of the habits you've developed, the choices and decisions you've made up to this point. If you're happy where you are, great. However, if you aren't, or if there is something you would like to improve, I'm here to tell you that this doesn't need to be your final destination. No matter how old you are or where you find yourself now, you have the choice to change – isn't that exciting?

In order to take back your life and start living the life you have always wanted, you must begin to get out of default mode – or what I call Groundhog Day mode – waking up and just repeating the previous day with no purpose or intensions. Life shouldn't be about going through the motions, but rather about continually evolving and growing. Those with winning attitudes and mindsets believe that life is about being intentional and purposeful in doing what you love.

I believe we all have been gifted with a set of incredibly unique of gifts, talents and skills – maybe you've been lucky to have already discovered yours. Each and every one of us has the power and ability to change our own life and others' lives for the better. I don't believe for a minute that you were created for anything but greatness. You were made to live a life filled with purpose, joy and fulfillment. Life is too short not to be living your best life. Life is too short not to be doing something that gets you out of bed in the morning with energy and something you call a passion. I was fortunate to have found mine early, but it is never too late.

No matter where you are in your life right now, no matter what might have happened in the past, I'm here to tell you that you have the power to change and redesign your life for the better. What is past is past; all that matters is today and this point forward. If you believe the future will be bright, it will, but you have to be willing to put in the work.

Every kid has a dream, but what unfortunately can happen, with the ebb and flow of life, is that over time they get pulled away from pursuing their dream due to either their own self-limiting beliefs or negative occurrences or even by what someone might have said to them. Maybe you can relate.

Understand that moving your life out of default mode takes courage, purpose, intention, and embracing the process (the mess). Change doesn't happen overnight. Don't be so busy running ragged that you don't take the necessary additional time to make a change that could benefit you. If this means stopping what you are currently doing so that you can make a real improvement, then do that, no matter how counterintuitive it feels. Bettering yourself in every way should be your highest priority.

Start by identifying what needs to be changed. The best thing is to take a piece of paper and a pen and start writing – the brain processes best when you put your thoughts on paper. Changes might include getting rid of certain people in your life, changing a job or a career, or even moving cities. It could be in one or many areas. The thing is that change won't happen unless you make it happen.

What you get out of life is a reflection of what you bring to it. That doesn't mean that life is fair, but if you don't like where you are, then make some changes. Today is another chance to become the person you know you can be. Measure your progress by being better than you were yesterday.

First decide what it is you really want. Reinvent your mindset. Recharge your body. Redesign your life. Recommit yourself to excellence every day.

It's never too late to

- Begin again
- Make a change
- Change those you hang out with
- Learn a new skill
- Change residence
- Change cities
- Help others
- Change your daily routine
- Make new friends
- Forgive yourself
- Choose happiness
- Have gratitude
- Set new goals
- Live your dreams

Your future self is begging you to make the commitment that you will thank yourself for one day.

If it doesn't challenge you,
it won't change you.

Chapter 48

A Winning Attitude Involves Forgiveness

Oprah Winfrey said, "True forgiveness is when you can say, 'Thank you for that experience.'" Wow! What an amazing attitude! The more life I experience, the more I realize that everything happens *for* us, not *to* us. Instead of playing the victim, we can choose to be the victor. But when it comes to forgiving others (or ourselves for that matter), it's easier said than done.

I believe that it's impossible to have a winner's attitude and mindset if you hold onto past grievances and grudges. It's impossible to have a winner's attitude and mindset if you have difficulty in forgiving others. When you hold grudges or are not willing to forgive others, you aren't only holding onto the past; worse, you are letting the past hold onto you. The most tragic thing of all is that when you hold onto the past, you can't fully embrace the future.

From the time we were little, our parents reminded us to forgive and forget. For me, it was especially my mother who repeated this mantra. But it's not easy. If we are told that letting go will bring peace of mind, we immediately respond with an archive of wrongs we have been subjected to. "Would you forgive such trespasses as easily if you were in my place?" we usually ask.

I've never met a person who hasn't been let down or hurt to some extent. It's a part of life – we all go through stuff that is unpleasant. I believe that moving on is important in acquiring a winner's attitude and mindset, because by holding on, the person you are hurting most is yourself. As hard as it is, if we don't forgive, we chain ourselves to a weight that we carry around with us every single day. Forgiveness has more to do with ourselves than with others. As soon as you decide to move on, you feel a sense of relief, and wonder why you didn't do it earlier.

Like everyone else, I have experienced my share of disappointments. Over time, I have experienced toxic relationships and failed business ventures, and I realize that holding onto grievances is counterproductive. For example, if you can't stop thinking or talking about how you were wronged, you become unpleasant company. And our not-so-tolerant world won't put up with that. In addition, if you spend your time judging those who've wronged you, you have no time for loving. You can't let this affect your path to excellence or to becoming a better person. You can let the world make you either bitter or better. Choose better.

Living in the past robs us of the beautiful present and a brighter future. Although forgiveness takes time, when you learn to forgive, you become a free person again. Today, you get to choose. Do you hold onto being a victim and prisoner of what's come before, or do you break the chains that are holding you back by forgiving and moving forward with a victor mentality? Choose to forgive.

When you forgive,
you in no way change the past –
but you sure do change the future.

– Bernard Meltzer

Chapter 49

The Road to Recovery Requires a Change in Attitude

After finishing my athletic career in duathlon at the age of 32, I can look back and be immensely proud of myself for achieving the goals I'd set and for reaching the top levels in my sport: two junior national titles, five world championships representing my country, one European championship, racing for four professional teams in Holland, France, Germany and Italy, and 53 race wins in over 15 countries. I knew deep in my heart I had gotten absolutely everything I could have out of my body and mind. By the end I was drained completely. With that in mind, I had zero regrets. OK, maybe one: I suppose I wish I had chosen a sport that had more money in it. The amount of work triathletes, duathletes and endurance athletes put in versus what they get back is pitiful. But I loved what I did, traveling the world and meeting so many amazing people along my journey.

In 2002, I decided to hang up the running shoes and the bike and to move to London to further my career in the fitness and sports industry. I had always known coaching and helping others was my destiny. I had big dreams and visions. However, after just three months of living in the United Kingdom, I began to fall into a deep state of depression. What I had envisioned wasn't panning out. I struggled to find the job I wanted, sometimes working as a cleaner or part-time fitness trainer for seven dollars an hour, and, as anyone who is familiar with rental prices in London would know, I was paying more for a studio room than I was earning per month. At one stage I had less than $200 in the bank. Another thing that weighed on me was the weather. All my life, growing up South Africa, I had been spoiled by being doused by the sun and vitamin D each day. I really believe that I'm solar powered!

Six months into my "new life" and after 13 years as a professional athlete, I was the lowest I'd ever been, mentally, emotionally and physically. I had dropped around 9 kilograms (around 20 pounds) in weight, and I was pale and incredibly fragile. I was unhappy, dejected and, yes, depressed. Now, if you can imagine, my weight during my racing and competitive days was around 62 kg (137 lbs.); I was now 53 kg (117 lbs.)! My muscles had severely deteriorated and disappeared in what seemed to be overnight! For the record, today I am a healthy 75 kg (165 lbs.).

It was on a phone call to my mother back to South Africa early one March morning when she gave me some of the most powerful advice I've ever received. Worried like any mother would be for her child, she told me, "Son, get up each morning, brush your hair and put on something nice. Then focus on what you are grateful for. Go out and be of service to someone else today. Even if it's helping an old lady with grocery bags cross the street or volunteering at the local YMCA." This is what she told me. She told me that I had to change my attitude if I wanted to change my circumstances and current situation. My mother then instructed me to write down just two or three things each evening that I had achieved that day, no matter how small.

Taking my mother's advice was the start of my recovery and road back to health and happiness. I also went on to take medication, which I was reluctant to do at first (of course – being a male with a large ego and a stubborn streak), and I felt my moods, energy and attitude change for the better. In fact, please, please, if you are suffering from depression, anorexia, bulimia, a mental illness, anything similar, get help! It is not a sign of weakness; in fact, asking for help is a sign of strength. Believe me, no matter how amazingly strong or successful you were or are, you can't do this alone. What is more encouraging than anything today is to see that more and more successful and publicly well-known people are coming out and talking about this challenge, especially men.

With athletes in the sports performance arena, I have witnessed that those who combine getting help with more positive outlooks and optimistic attitudes recover and return to play much more quickly than those who don't. Athletes who focus on what they *can do*, instead of what they *can't do*, heal way more quickly. Athletes who bemoan their bad luck and complain about how unfortunate they are take way longer to get back to full fitness. I recall a chat I had with South African rugby international Jesse Kriel in April 2019. Jesse had just torn ligaments in a game playing for the Blue Bulls. I messaged him to say what bad luck it was and to stay positive. I also asked him if he felt he had any chance of being ready for the World Cup in Japan, which was happening only a few weeks later. At the time he was lying in hospital in Pretoria after an operation, and to be honest I thought he'd be bitter and bemoaning his bad luck. But Jesse was getting medical aid and advice. His reply showed me just how champion minded he is. His text said, "Attitude is everything, and with some hard work on my rehab, I'll be back ready to play." And indeed he was. The South African rugby team won the World Cup in Japan and Jesse was part of the victorious squad!

You see, it's all a choice. Champions see setbacks as wonderful opportunities for even better comebacks. Taking into account the importance and benefits of medicine, I do strongly believe that a more positive attitude and mindset speed up the healing process.

Taking charge of what occupies your mind and reevaluating the way you think can improve your physical health and well-being.

Chapter 50

Winners Embrace Change

English theoretical physicist and professor Stephen Hawking famously said, "Intelligence is the ability to adapt to change." My experience shows this to be true. The most successful people I've met are those who are able to keep a great attitude, stay open-minded – and adapt to change. They have the mindset that views change as growth.

In life, there is only one thing that's constant, and that is change. Nothing is permanent. I can promise you this: If you aren't OK with change or being uncomfortable sometimes, you will never make the most of your potential and talents. You will never be able to reach the greatness you have within. If you're not willing to adapt to change, you will always hold yourself back from becoming the best you can be.

A winning attitude involves embracing change, but the thought of making a change, be it big or small, can sometimes be an intimidating one. One reason is that we are afraid we might lose something that either we already have or we have invested much time and energy in. But you can't expect something to improve if fear keeps you stuck in the same old thought patterns. It would be a tragedy to let fear stop you from living your life to its full potential. I've always had the belief that I'd rather try and fail than be 70 years of age and wonder what might have been if I had made different choices and hadn't let fear or discomfort get in my way.

However, change can be scary. Change can be hard, confusing and messy – whether it's within your career, your team, your home or your relationships. But we must embrace it in order to continue to grow. The thing with change is that although you may lose something good, you may also gain something better. Even if it seems that your life has changed for the worse, there is always some sort of good that can be found when life takes a different turn. Also, remember that not all positive change feels positive in the beginning. In fact in most cases it's the opposite. The key is to trust yourself and embrace the process.

If you stay in your comfort zone all your life and never welcome change, it will be difficult if not impossible to grow as a person, to learn from mistakes, and to become the best self you can be. If you don't like where you are in life right now, then consider your best change options.

You are never too old to set a new dream, goal or vision. You are never too old to change the direction you were once heading. You are never stuck. When traveling and speaking around the world, I meet so many people who are unhappy or unfulfilled, who tell me they've been in the same line of work for 30 years and they can't change now. Sounding almost defeated, they tell me it's too late. But there is no limit to how many times you can reinvent yourself.

What does it look like to not let fear get in the way? It looks like a 56-year-old woman named Moira. I was speaking in Los Angeles last year, and during the break I got to meet Moira, who had been in sales and marketing for most of her life. She said she'd always wanted to be involved in the fitness industry as her passion was to help others improve their lifestyles. Long story short, she quit her job, took an online course to become a wellness coach, and is now consulting and training clients. She decided to take on the winner's attitude and take that leap. I spoke with her a few weeks back and she told me that she's happier than ever. Her only regret was not making that change sooner!

Not letting fear get in the way also looks like me. A few years ago, after spending over two decades in the fitness industry, I felt that I'd become stale and unmotivated, and that it was time for a change in life. I had dedicated myself to becoming one of the best trainers in the performance sector. However, I had gotten to a stage where I was no longer fueled by what I once called my passion, and it was beginning to affect my relationships, health and happiness. I knew I needed a change.

Being in the profession of encouraging others to embrace change and to get uncomfortable, I asked myself if I was practicing what I preached and if I was ready to make the change. I knew that I needed to redesign my life with a new passion and purpose. I'd always loved helping and seeing others excel, and I felt the calling to write and speak on culture, team dynamics and leadership. I had to relearn, re-brand and remarket myself over a period of many years. I had to learn to get uncomfortable again; I had to take risks and leave behind what I was so comfortable with and so well known for. I took the leap of faith, and now 1,000 paid talks, over 100,000 people reached, more than 50 countries visited, numerous TV appearances and four books later, the rest, as they say, is history.

What about you? Are you happy where you are right now? If not, what's holding you back from making a change? If you are stuck on old stories and old beliefs, the ones that fill you with self-doubt and worry, you will never be what this world needs. Are you afraid to let go of your comfort zone? How will you know how amazing you could have become if you never let go? If not now, when?

Go on; it's time to give up the good for the great. You deserve it! This world needs your best self. Progress involves constant change. Happiness involves change. You were not placed on this earth to be average or mediocre. You deserve to be happy and fulfilled. The change might be scary at first, but trust the process, and more importantly trust in yourself every day.

You were made for greatness, so what are you waiting for?

Everyone thinks of changing the world,
but no one thinks of changing himself.

– Leo Tolstoy

Conclusion

As we close, I commend you for taking the time to read this book. You now have the valuable tools to help you develop a winning attitude and mindset. Choose to use them. This requires spending time – just as with establishing any other skill – and putting in the daily work and staying consistent. It is both doable and lifelong rewarding.

We have discussed a broad spectrum of steps and strategies that you can put into practice. Be patient with yourself. You will have days along the way where you feel like a failure, but that's normal. Believe in yourself and stay the journey. You are your most valuable investment.

Let's review the simple yet profound ways we covered to help you develop a positive attitude and mindset.

Take control of your thoughts. Avoid people who bring you down, and be your own greatest fan. Never lower your standards to please someone else.

Remember that a positive mental attitude is indeed the best secret weapon you can have. Let others see your positivity and potential. Learn from your failures (the sources of some of the most important lessons) and celebrate your victories, big and small.

Employ your Attitude Police to stop negative thoughts and steer you to positive ones. Focus on being the best YOU you can be. View stresses as opportunities to show your stuff. Let go of the burdens of the past and let optimism guide you.

Use intentional and consistent self-discipline. It is a must if you are to achieve your goals. Be the standout who gives the extra 5% that others don't.

Think about the role models we talked about. They set the example of brightening others' days and staying positive in spite of negative odds. Work with enthusiasm every day, and never let those who refuse to see your potential destroy it.

Consider the ways that empathy makes a difference in life. Get to know and accept your own qualities and flaws; it helps you accept the qualities and flaws in others. Build and nurture those relationships with empathy and kindness. Use your self-awareness to get along better with others and to succeed.

Practicing gratitude, appreciation, and self-reflection (GAS) every day gives you perspective and helps you identify your greater purpose and vision. Recognize that no one has all the answers, and respect the ideas of others so that they will be interested in respecting yours.

Embrace change that improves who and what you are. While it is important to retain one's values, people who are unwilling to consider new ideas will be left behind. Commit each day to outdoing yesterday. Adding forgiveness and gratitude to your life will influence it in wonderful and unforeseeable ways.

I recently heard a story about two friends I'll call Bob and Ray who met one evening for a drink. Bob had asked Ray whether it was too late to start medical school; after all, he wouldn't be hanging out his shingle until he was 48. Ray asked Bob if he would want to be a doctor when he turned 48, so Bob chose to take the leap and go to med school. That was eight years earlier. Their meeting this evening was to toast Bob's new practice.

Likewise time will pass in your life. Pick any number of weeks, months, or years. At that point do you want to be living up to your potential? Do you want to have succeeded far beyond what you gave yourself credit for? Then choose consistent daily action. Choose consistent daily self-discipline.

I encourage you to keep going no matter what. Yes, there will be obstacles and challenges, but choose to believe in the future and to think positive thoughts. Know that you already have everything you need within you; now it's time to work on becoming the very best version of you. Choose to commit each day to developing the attitude and mindset that will set you up to positively transform you career, your relationships and your life.

Your future self is waiting to thank you.
– Allistair

A great attitude becomes a great day,
Which becomes a great week,
Which becomes a great month,
Which becomes a great year,
Which becomes a great life.

Appendix

10 Daily Practices to Create a Winning Mindset and Attitude

1. Wake up with *gratitude*
2. Have a *game plan* for the day
3. Get around *good people*
4. *Read* everyday
5. Practice *emotional intelligence*
6. Spend your day in *appreciation*
7. *Exercise* and hydrate
8. See challenges as *opportunities*
9. Nurture *relationships*
10. *Self-reflect* at the end of each day

25 Habits of People with a Winning Attitude and Mindset

1. They smile more
2. They listen to first understand, not reply
3. They stay accountable to themselves and others
4. They stay positive and optimistic
5. They treat others in the same way they want to be treated
6. They avoid arguments or heated discussions
7. They can laugh at themselves
8. They have empowering self-talk
9. They are confident, yet have a sense of humility
10. They don't push their beliefs on others
11. They don't gossip about others
12. They apologize (and don't view it as a sign of weakness)
13. They don't seek (or need) your approval
14. They are mindful of others
15. They show appreciation for others
16. They uphold a healthy set of boundaries
17. They aren't afraid to give genuine praise to others
18. They don't complain or blame
19. They don't judge
20. They are happy for other people's success
21. They create meaningful relationships
22. They keep open-minded
23. They stay consistent in their moods
24. They have empathy
25. They practice gratitude

Having a vision for your life provides these 5 benefits

1. It gives meaning and purpose to what you're doing
2. It provides clarity
3. It gives meaning and purpose to what you're doing
4. It motivates you through challenging times
5. It provides validation and the feeling of profound accomplishment when you succeed

6 Questions to Help You Discover Your Vision

1. What is close to your heart and really matters to you in life?
2. What would bring you more joy in your life?
3. What do you really care about?
4. What are your talents? What's special about you?
5. What would you like to have more of in your life?
6. What legacy would you like to leave behind?

3 Factors in the Gap between Where You Are Now and Where You Want to Be

1. The amount of time and work you're willing to put in
2. The level of belief you have in yourself
3. Your ability to overcome adversity and failure, and learn from it

Make These Mantras a Part of Your Vocabulary

I can

I will

I believe

I have what it takes

All things are possible

5 Ways to Distance Yourself from Negativity

1. Unfollow and delete negative people and platforms on social media

2. Don't spend a lot of time watching or listening to the news on TV or radio

3. Distance yourself from the energy vampires

4. Don't entertain gossip

5. Don't get into discussions about politics or religion

Helpful Hints to a Better Relationship with Yourself

- Practice gratitude and appreciation

- Be good to yourself

- Refrain from judging others and yourself

- Learn to see the good in yourself and others

- Love and accept who you are right now

- Let go of the past; it's gone

- Forgive yourself and others

- Self-reflect daily; write things down

- Wake up each morning and tell yourself how awesome you really are!

Spend time with people who are

- Able to get things done
- Appreciative
- Authentic
- Consistent
- Empathetic
- Generous
- Going places
- Grateful
- Happy for others' success
- Helpful
- Honest
- Humble
- Inspiring
- Not judgmental
- On a mission
- Positive
- Purposeful
- Selfless
- Sincere
- There for you
- Uplifting

5 Ss When Approaching or Meeting Someone

1. Smile on approaching the person
2. Shake hands (always look them in the eye)
3. Share a compliment (it can be anything, even "I love your shoes!")
4. Share your contact information (have a business card ready)
5. Send a follow-up within 48 hours (a text or an e-mail to say that it was a pleasure to meet them)

5 Regrets Expressed by the Dying

1. I wish I'd had the courage to live a life true to myself, not the life others expected of me.
2. I wish I hadn't worked so much.
3. I wish I'd had the courage to express my feelings.
4. I wish I had stayed in touch with my friends.
5. I wish that I had let myself be happier.

10 Ways to Increase Your Joy and Happiness

1. Be grateful
2. Give of your time, and help others
3. Appreciate the small things in life more
4. Enjoy the company of those you love
5. Be more accepting of yourself
6. Watch your favorite show or a great comedy
7. Improve your self-talk
8. Do more of the things you love to do
9. Take care of your health
10. Do not take yourself so seriously

9 Ways to Invest in Yourself

1. Read more
2. Exercise – hire a trainer
3. Listen to podcasts
4. Watch interesting documentaries, TED talks or educational programs
5. Go to workshops/seminars
6. Study or enroll in a new course
7. Speak to different people in different sectors and industries
8. Take someone you can learn from out for coffee or lunch
9. Find a mentor/coach in the area you want to get better at

Learning how and when to say no helps you to

- free up more time to do the things you want to do or need to do.

- choose what does and what doesn't fit with your greater vision and purpose.

- realize what you simply don't enjoy doing anymore.

- face the fact that with some people it's always a take-take. It's important to say no to people who don't support you, people who might manipulate you, people who are always in some way using you. Making this decision also helps you find the win-win relationships that boost your quality of life. Those people who are always taking eventually drain your soul and make you feel bad.

- notice what is colliding or running into more important things in your life, like family commitments and other priorities.

3 Ways to Effectively Say No

1. Step up and just say it
2. Be firm and be selfish in the appropriate way
3. Set boundaries

You demonstrate signs that you have high emotional intelligence when you

- smile more
- forgive more
- have patience
- listen to understand, not to reply
- remember people's names
- don't interrupt others
- don't respond to negativity
- are able to control your anger
- are grateful and have empathy
- are respectful and have manners
- respect differences and other opinions
- don't gossip about others
- gather all the facts first
- don't judge quickly
- show appreciation
- are open-minded
- prefer to be silent than to engage in drama
- are interested in others more than yourself

4 Tips to Become a More Empathetic Person

1. Listen more than you speak

2. Don't make assumptions

3. Challenge yourself to see things from the other person's view

4. Welcome feedback

5 Benefits of Staying Open-minded

1. You are more approachable to others

2. You are more empathetic

3. You are viewed as someone worth listening to because your ideas are seen as well thought out

4. Your likeability increases because you are open to listening

5. You open yourself up to learning more

It's never too late to

- begin again
- make a change
- change those you hang out with
- learn a new skill
- relocate
- help others
- change your daily routine
- move cities
- choose happiness
- live your dreams
- set new goals
- forgive yourself
- have gratitude
- make new friends

3 Questions to Ask Yourself at the End of the Day

1. What did I do well today?
2. What could I have done better today?
3. Who did I make better today?

More about Allistair McCaw

An inspiring, passionate and highly motivated speaker, Allistair has positively impacted the mindsets, performances, cultures, and lives of thousands of people around the world. Driven by his deeper purpose and vision, he has been able to share his knowledge, wisdom, and vast experience working with some of the world's best performers in their fields.

Why not book Allistair for your next conference, speaking or team event? Allistair consults and presents on these topics:

- Leadership

- Team Culture

- Self-development

- Becoming Champion Minded

Allistair also works as a one-on-one professional coach in all of these fields.

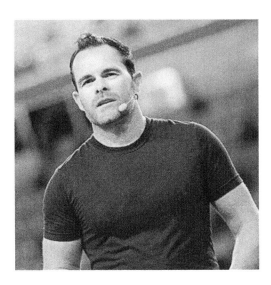

For more details and customized pricing,

please contact Allistair at

mccawmethod@gmail.com

Follow Allistair on social media!

Twitter: @allistairmccaw

Instagram: BeChampionMinded

Facebook: Allistair McCaw Page

Hashtag on all social media: #WinningAttitudeMindsetBook

www.allistairmccaw.com

All books available on Amazon.com

About Denise McCabe

Denise McCabe is a freelance nonfiction editor. She has been helping writers shape, polish, and perfect their writing since 2002. Denise also develops and facilitates seminars in business writing and email effectiveness.

Denise works with:

- Authors / Subject matter experts
- Corporations
- Government agencies
- Associations
- Educational institutions
- Banking institutions

For more details, please contact:

denise@mccabeediting.com

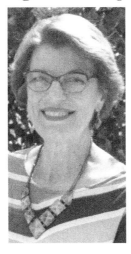

---

*Your attitude can be your best friend or
your worst enemy,
and each day you get to choose that.*

– Herm Edwards

Printed in Great Britain
by Amazon

25547567R00129